THIS BOOK MAY SAVE YOUR LIFE...

Every new idea goes through three phases:

Phase 1: It is ignored...

Phase 2: It is ridiculed...

Phase 3: The Establishment claims it as their own discovery.

Forty years ago wholistic medical practitioners were warning that smoking was a major precursor of cancer. The orthodox medical and governmental establishments possessed the same facts and information, yet for twenty-five years they not only withheld this information but actually financed studies to prove smoking was non-injurious.

Only since 1960 has the American Cancer Society, along with the governmental, industrial and medical complex, admitted what prevention-minded health professionals were shouting all along. Timidly, grudgingly at first, and now — **as if they had discovered it** — they campaign that smoking is bad for your health.

For many years nutritionally-knowledgeable health professionals have recognized that cancer and its prevention can be nutritionally controlled. Orthodox medicine has continually rejected and ridiculed any nutritional cause of cancer. Finally, in 1982, the prestigious **National Academy of Science has published a report recognizing the vital connection of diet to cancer cause and prevention.**

In its own report, however, the N.A.S. states that it will take *twenty years*, or more, to formulate these findings into a practical application! As with smoking, can you wait twenty years to apply this nutritional information to prevent or control cancer malignancy?

This book presents, in understandable detail, the discoveries and cancer prevention information contained in the National Academy of Science report, together with practical application and implementation to put this undeniably correct nutrition information to work for you **NOW**, not twenty years from now.

Most of the 365,000 Americans who will become cancer victims this year could have remained cancer free, or at least controlled their disease, with the information contained in this book.

Nutrition: The Cancer Answer is the result of twelve years of vigorous research by a well-known author in the field of health and cancer prevention.

Nutrition: The Cancer Answer will:

1. Give you the research-based proof that cancer can be prevented and controlled.
2. Rid you of the fear of ever contracting cancer in your lifetime.
3. Present carefully researched studies of various societies which enjoy cancer-free lives.
4. Show you how you can enjoy exuberant good health untouched by the *1 in 3 cancer epidemic*. Included is a "Gourmet Guide" to cancer prevention filled with easy and delicious recipes for vibrant good health.

Nutrition:
The Cancer Answer

by
Maureen Kennedy Salaman, M.Sc.

STATFORD PUBLISHING
Menlo Park, California

Library of Congress No. 83-61514
ISBN: 0-913087-01-7

Original Hardcover Edition, June, 1983
First Paperback Edition, September, 1984
Seventh Printing, November, 1988

Published by
Statford Publishing
1259 El Camino Real, Suite 1500
Menlo Park, CA 94025

Printed in The United States of America

DEDICATION

To Connie and Ronn Haus
whose inspiration feeds the souls
of millions, including mine; and
to Shirley and Ken Foreman,
who are the salt of the earth who
preserve and sustain.

ACKNOWLEDGMENTS
Salt Talks

Matthew 5:13 says, "Ye are the salt of the earth but if the salt has lost its savor, how will you be preserved? It is, thenceforth, good for nothing but to be cast out and trodden underfoot of men."

Many times a great nation is preserved and sustained by a small remnant of people, a small group of individualists who stand in the gap in the hour of crisis. George Washington was relying heavily on that remnant when he said, "Let none but Americans stand guard tonight."

If America is to be preserved, it will be through this remnant. I have renewed hope for our great nation because this remnant is visible to me in the form of many individuals, too numerous to list them all. They are the unsung heroes and heroines, the quiet men and women of deep conviction who do the world's work and bear the world's weight on their shoulders and live brilliantly in the depths of the soul. These people know that the reward of genius may be the gold medal or the cup of hemlock.

These are the salt of the earth that has not lost its savor. They are the light that shines in the darkness. They are the heroes through whom truth and right endure.

I have great hope, for I know many of them: Ken and Hazel Kidwell, Al and Lilly Battista, Betty Lee Morales, John T. Clark, Carol and Rodger Mehrtens, Paul Virgin, Kurt Donsbach, Greg and Karen Kaye, Andrew McNaughton, Glen Rutherford, Dr. Robert Mendelsohn, Fred Blahut, Mike Blair, Willis Carto, Hal and Linda Card, Linda Wick, Peggy MacDonald, Mrs. Basset, John Fink, Gene Arceri, Kim and Kerry Asay, Earl Irons, Sam and Judy Goeltz, Dorothy Hart, Floyd Weston, Don Picket, Louie Popp, Karl Rolfes, and the many more unnamed thousands of you who sustain and preserve our greatness as a people.

I wish to express special thanks to Dr. Kurt Donsbach for the material in Chapter Five regarding the digestive system and to Bill Koester and Al Mason, whose scalpel-like editing of the manuscript strengthened the words that remain.

iv

TABLE OF CONTENTS

Introduction

Etched in the memories of generation after generation, Dickens' "It was the best of times; it was the worst of times" stamps "A Tale of Two Cities" as an eternal marker of a major historical shift. Similarly, the Federalist Papers and the Declaration of Independence are the literary symbols of the rise of a new social order out of the destruction of its predecessor.

Now, author Maureen Salaman, employing the scientific research of Harold Manner and other eminent scientists, has produced this outstanding literary standard, destined to mark the end of the dark age of medical oppression and the beginning of the new era of health freedom.

Her historical critique of the moral bankruptcy of the high priests of modern medicine guarantees this work a secure position alongside the classical documentations of medical deceit, beginning with Koestler's "Case of the Midwife Toad" and extending through a fifty-year period to Joseph Hixon's "The Patchwork Mouse."

Indeed, the clarity of the Salaman dissertation embarrasses anyone — and certainly me — who ever bought into modern medicine's outrageous belief system.

And the safe and sane Salaman presription offers hope based on rational thought and optimism founded on fundamental principles of human history.

Modern medicine's death-oriented tyranny results from a disastrous rejection of belief in nutrition — in favor of prostitution to the "better living through chemistry" approach, a pathway which directly led to the modern iatrogenic epidemics of cancer, heart disease and stroke.

In contrast, this landmark work offers us the recipe — and the recipes — for health, for life, and for human survival. I emphasize the words "human survival" because modern medicine poses an overwhelming threat, not only to individual lives, but to life itself.

Nutrition — the Cancer Answer appears just in time to rescue us, personally and nationally, from the iatrogenicide perpetuated by the idolatrous priesthood of the Religion of Modern Medicine. Maureen Salaman merits our deepest gratitude.

Robert S. Mendelsohn, M.D.

PART I:
Foreword

Cancer Prevention And Alleviation In Our Lifetime

If you are impressed by statistics you will find it interesting that more than a million Americans who were alive when this book was begun, and might have benefited from it, will never read it. Or even hear of it. They are dead — victims of mankind's most vicious degenerative disease: Cancer.

Tragic? Yes. But no more ironic than the fact that the medical philosophy on which this book is based could have saved perhaps half of those lives — and prevented most of the victims from ever contracting cancer in the first place. It is called preventive medicine. To some, it is known as metabolic, or holistic, medicine. (Or wholistic, thus to avoid a religious connotation and identify it more properly with the whole-being concept of wellness and natural healing espoused by its practitioners and proponents.)

By whatever name, the preventive approach to combating cancer is what this book is all about. And nothing states its basic premise more succinctly than the wise old adage, "An ounce of prevention is worth a pound of cure." Which is not to say that cancer is controllable only by preventing it; even for those who do contract it, cancer can be reversed — and this book will offer proof of that assertion. More important, however, is that you, as a potential statistic, learn *now* how to deny cancer a foothold or future in your life. To slam the door on it. To beat it, as this book tells you how.

Cancer is usually accompanied by a secondary, undiagnosed metabolic dysfunction. In almost all cases, only a skilled physician using the consortium of diagnostic and therapeutic tools at his command is capable of programming and supervising a complete regimen to overcome or reverse this malignancy. The information within these pages is not meant, therefore, to be a primer for self-treatment of an already entrenched degenerative disease.

What this book does include is a doctor's protocol for treatment. It is intended to serve principally as both an outline and an explanation, to the prospective patient, of the metabolic physician's general procedure. This does not preclude the implementation, by those of us who are well, of a proven prevention program as detailed in the chapters to follow. When adhered to in conjunction with the normal health care advice of a holistic physician and/or nutritionist, it will prevent you or a loved one from becoming a victim of this most devastating of diseases. At the heart of this program are two simple but all-important essentials: natural foods and supplemental nutrition in the form of vitamins and minerals.

The program you will learn about in this book is specifically addressed to cancer prevention. Its effectiveness is based on the addition or restoration to the diet of a daily intake of those nutrients and foods that have heretofore been neglected in otherwise good nutritional programs. Its applicability is not contraindicated by any but the most unique metabolic diseases. Best of all, it is a diet that can be added to or integrated with all otherwise nutritionally-adequate regimens.

Conventional medicine is only now just beginning to investigate the relationship between nutrition and cancer. While this beginning is certainly welcome and long overdue, it will be many years before the medical establishment in general will finally be forced to accept the realities that have been known to the health movement for so long and which are described in the pages of this book. With Americans dying from cancer at the rate of 400,000 a year, we can ill afford to wait 10 or 20 years for orthodox medicine to re-invent the wheel before applying what is already known about nutrition and cancer in our daily lives.

As this book was about to go to press, the Committee on Diet, Nutrition and Cancer of the prestigious National Research Council (the principal operating agency of the National Academy of Sciences) released a preliminary report of its findings about the relationship between cancer and nutrition. This research was commissioned in June, 1980, by the National Cancer Institute (NCI). Actually, NCI had commissioned two reports on the subject. The first was merely to determine whether there were any evidence to link cancer with nutrition and diet. The second was to suggest directions for future research along these lines.

The National Research Council (NRC) assigned the task to the executive office of its Assembly of Life Sciences (ALS), which created a 13-member committee with experts from the fields of biochemistry, microbiology, embryology, epidemiology, experimental oncology, internal medicine, microbial genetics, molecular biology, molecular genetics, nutrition, nutrition education, public health and toxicology. This blue-ribbon panel did not study or evaluate nutrition in relation to cancer therapy but only addressed itself to diet and nutrition in relation to the cause and prevention of cancer. After two years of labor, this is what the experts found and published late in 1982:

"It has become absolutely clear that cigarettes are the cause of approximately one quarter of all the fatal cancers in the United States. If the population had been persuaded to stop smoking when the association with lung cancer was first reported, these cancer deaths would not now be occurring. Twenty years ago the 'stop smoking' message required some rather cautious wording. Today, the facts are clear, and the choice of words is not so important.... The public is now asking about the causes of cancers that are not associated with smoking.... We are in an interim stage of knowledge similar to that for cigarettes 20 years ago. Therefore, in the judgement of the committee, it is now the time to offer some interim guidelines on diet and cancer."

In other words, to read between the lines, it may be another 20 years before orthodox medicine is as willing to admit the relationship between diet and cancer as they are now willing to admit the relationship between smoking cigarettes and cancer. A report issued by Drs. Eon McDonald and Henry Garland on behalf of the California Medical Association, as late as 1953, assured the public that smoking a pack of cigarettes a day was "a harmless pass time". We do not find doctors saying such things today. They have come a long way, baby. But can we wait another 20 years to apply the rules of sound nutrition in the battle against cancer while hundreds of thousands of people die for lack of knowledge? The only humane answer is a resounding "Absolutely not!"

It would be yet another year, the NRC Committee said in its first report, before publication of its recommendations for future research. How many more years before funding is obtained for that research, the research itself is done, the conclusions, if any, published, the committee's report did not even speculate. And after publication of the results of the research on diet and cancer, how many further years are to elapse as the old school of thought about cancer treatment battles stubbornly with the new?

Some highlights relative to this whole issue taken from the NRC report are as follow:

1. "The Committee concluded that the differences in the rates at which various cancers occur in different human populations are often correlated with differences in diet. The likelihood that some of these correlations reflect causality is strengthened by laboratory evidence that similar dietary patterns and components of food also affect the incidence of certain cancers in animals."

2. "In general, the evidence suggests that some types of diets and some dietary components tend to increase the risk of cancer, whereas others tend to decrease it."

The Committee made some tentative conclusions as to which dietary elements were associated with cancer development and which were associated with cancer prevention. These conclusions were consistent with the detailed discussions of various dietary factors you will encounter in the following pages.

Futher evidence of the growing awareness about the relationship between nutrition and cancer was the article entitled "Diet Studies" in the *The Wall Street Journal* Nov. 15, 1982, which reported there was a growing amount of evidence that vitamins A, C, E, Beta Carotene and the mineral selenium may block the process by which the body's cells turn malignant. *The Wall Street Journal* reported on the work of Dr. Seymour L. Romney at Albert Einstein College of Medicine in New York, who found that women suffering from pre-cancerous changes of the cervix consumed on the average less vitamins C and A and Beta Carotene than women who did not have those changes. And it reported on the work of Dr. Frank L. Meyskens Jr. and his team at the University of Arizona which showed the application of retinoids (Vitamin A) to pre-cancerous cells in the cervix caused six cases of remission out of 18 patients after only four days of treatment.

The Wall Street Journal article also reports on a Beta Carotene study at Harvard in which 20,000 doctors will test on themselves over the next five years the efficacy of Beta Carotene (essentially Vitamin A) as a cancer preventative. Again, we are looking at years of study to get results. Years in which thousands of patients of these same 20,000 doctors may die for want of the same treatment their doctors are taking in an experiment.

If each year of delay in the application of what we already know about the relationship between cancer and nutrition is to result in 400,000 dead Americans, then we cannot wait 20 years and 8,000,000 dead Americans for orthodox science to recognize about nutrition and cancer what is already known about cigarettes and cancer. We cannot wait five years for 10,000 doctors out of 20,000 in the Harvard study to develop cancer because they are taking a placebo instead of Vitamin A, because that is 2,000,000 dead cancer patients. And if you happen to be one of the 400,000 Americans who will die of cancer in the next year, we cannot even wait the one year it will take for the National Research Council to get around to issuing its suggestions for further research. We must use what we know about cancer and diet and let the medical journals catch up later. To this purpose this book is written.

CHAPTER 1:

The Catastrophe of Cancer

"When the Air Force is trying to sell bombers, it uses every trick of the advertising trade. Well, all right, we have to do that too. Of course, it's inevitable when you go to the public for money."

M.B. Shimkin, M.D., National Cancer
Institute and author of **Science and Cancer**
(U.S. Dept. of Health, Education & Welfare)

During one month of each year (April) nearly every family in the U.S. will be called on by an American Cancer Society (ACS) volunteer. They will be asked to contribute money to "fight cancer with a check-up and a check," according to the society's favorite slogan. Reinforced by a sophisticated multimedia campaign and a proclamation by the President declaring April "Cancer Control Month," this unprecedented mobilization stands to gross the ACS $150 million.

When it was founded in 1913, the ACS described itself as a "temporary" organization; it would cease to exist once cancer had been eradicated. Seven decades later, the Society is the richest private charity in the world. And cancer is more of a problem than ever before! In the past 10 years alone, during which the ACS collected more than $1 billion from the cancer-phobic American public, the cancer death rate climbed 12 percent.

According to one disgruntled volunteer, the ACS has become "a self-perpetuating vested interest" and "a very profitable one" for many of those involved. In 1979, the National Information Bureau (NIB), a respected independent charity-watchdog organization, listed the ACS among the groups which do not meet its standards. Nonetheless, the ACS has consistently been the loudest voice of the cancer establishment, and today it remains entrenched in the front lines of the government's war on cancer.

Like the other large bureaucracies of the health care delivery system, the ACS is not representative of the public at large. Many of its directors and members of its various scientific committees have direct financial links to chemical industries and drug companies; its medical advisors, meanwhile, are drawn exclusively from the fields of orthodox cancer treatment (i.e., surgery, radiation, and chemotherapy). Not surprisingly, the society advocates treating cancer rather than preventing it. To this day the only hazards it warns people about are cigarettes and alcohol. The many other processes and products shown to trigger a majority of human cancers, such as chemical and industrial pollution, drugs like DES, radiation, junk food, and food additives are ignored. (In 1977 the ACS adopted a "pro-saccharin stand" after receiving a large grant from a major cola company, which is also a substantial contributor to the Calorie Control Council, the official name of the saccharin lobby.)

In addition to its anti-prevention and pro-industry stance, the ACS, according to its critics, spends its lavish budget improperly, blacklisting promising original research that is not confined to avenues predetermined by its own staff and grant procedures.

ACS executives loudly proclaim that the ACS "is a people-benefit kind of organization with by far the major proportion of its resources spent for caring and rehabilitating the cancer patient." An analysis of ACS' 1978 budget, however, reveals that only $6.2 million, or 5 percent, went to "assistance to individual patients." Grants for research, meanwhile, amounted to $35.6 million, or 27 percent of the Society's spending that year. At $44 million, the salaries and benefits for ACS' paid staff of 3,000 people (quite large for a "volunteer organization" which conducts no research of its own!) exceeded the Society's expenditures for research and patient care put together. By far the largest proportion of the 1978 ACS budget, $74 million, or 56 percent, went toward the

Society's own administrative and office expenses, fund raising, rent, office supplies, postage. Incredibly, more than $10,000 a day was spent for telephone calls.[1]

The ACS also lobbies vigorously to suppress new ideas within the medical community, where it wields tremendous power. Science journalist Robert Houston explained how the process works. "Independent, unconventional research," he noted, "tends to be blocked by the actions of the ACS, by their whole system of blacklisting and vilification of new therapies. ACS maintains an official blacklist, *Unproven Methods of Cancer Management*, 'unproven' being their code word for 'quack.' Once you are on this list, it is very difficult, if not impossible, to get off; it is like trying to get out of hell. And some of the most promising things in cancer research have landed on that list."[2]

Among the many reputable researchers and clinicians summarily blacklisted by ACS are the late Max Gerson, M.D. (of whom Dr. Albert Schweitzer wrote, "I see in him one of the most eminent geniuses in the history of medicine"); Andrew Ivy, M.D., Ph.D. (former vice president of the University of Illinois); and Ernst Krebs, Jr., Ph.D., (the co-discoverer of Laetrile and vitamin B15). In *The Cancer Syndrome* (Grove, 1980), Ralph Moss, Ph.D., documents how official sources of funding dry up for blacklisted individuals. Not surprisingly, the unconventional approaches are rarely tested. As Houston emphasized, "It should be noted that 'unproven' is not synonymous with 'disproven'."[3]

It seems incredible that an organization such as the ACS, established to champion new cancer research, should in fact spend much of its budget actively *suppressing* new ideas.

Cancer: A Modern Medicine Phenomenon

Cancer was recorded by the early Greeks and from time to time throughout European history. In 1764, Johann Philip published a treatise, at Frankfurt am Main, attributing cancer to an excess of acidic substances in food and drink. The earliest statistical evidence (as opposed to scattered reporting) was probably

4 NUTRITION THE CANCER ANSWER

collected by the Registrar General of England and Wales for the period between 1838 and 1859. The death rate of approximately 20 per 100,000 noted at that time was not significant and certainly no greater than from many other diseases.

During the late 19th Century it became evident to many medical observers that cancer was on the increase throughout the world, especially in the industrialized parts of Europe and North America. This increase exploded in the 20th Century — not, however, as the result of improved medical diagnosis or more accurate collection and interpretation of statistical evidence; the increase in cancer was *real,* as Chart 1 shows.

Chart 1 **Percent Change In Cancer Deaths By Decade** **United States 1900 - 1979**			
Date	Deaths from Cancer	Increase from previous decade	Percent increase per decade
1900	41,000		
1910	65,000	+24,000	+58.54%
1920	85,000	+20,000	+30.77%
1930	118,000	+33,000	+38.82%
1940	158,000	+40,000	+33.90%
1950	211,000	+53,000	+33.54%
1960	260,047	+49,047	+23.24%
1970	330,700	+70,653	+27.16%
1980	405,000	+74,300 (est.)	+22.46%

In 1900 only 41,000 Americans died of cancer. Since 1900 every decade has seen a gigantic 23 to 60 percent increase in the death rate.

In 1980 well over 400,000 Americans died of cancer, which is the only major cause of death that has continued to increase from 1900 to the present time. Whereas the death rate from cancer was 64 per 100,000 persons in 1900, today it is over 170. More people now die of cancer each year in the United States than the combined fatalities of the Korean and Vietnamese wars. Worse, the death rates from cancer are still increasing, and more people are dying of cancer at an early age than at any time in the history of the world.[4]

The multi-billion-dollar "war on cancer" instituted by President Richard Nixon in the early 1970s focused only on use of orthodox treatments by the medical establishments: surgery, radiation and chemotherapy — the cut, burn and poison approach which has, to the present, failed to provide a solution. The result of this political and medical inertia has been a continuation of the disastrous increase in cancer deaths since the early 1970s (see Chart 2 on page 6).

When the final tabulation is completed, the American Cancer Society estimates the deaths from breast cancer will have been 106,900 in 1979 (compared to 88,700 in 1975) and 112,000 for lung cancer in 1979 (compared to 91,000 in 1975)[5]. This continually increasing escalation of cancer incidence should have changed the tunnel-vision science of the medical establishment, but no sign of change is evident.

In addition, there has been little change in the five-year survival rate for cancer since 1955. A slight statistical improvement from the 1930s to 1955 can be attributed to improvements in operating room procedures rather than to cancer research, i.e., the introduction of antibiotics and blood transfusions that have enabled more patients to survive cancer operations. Since 1955 the cancer survival rate has flattened out as the benefits from improved procedures were absorbed.

Orthodox Treatment of Cancer

Cancer statistics in the U.S. yield one irrefutable conclusion: the incidence of cancer is increasing. At the same time the rate of expenditure on cancer research is also increasing and has been throughout this century (see Chart 3 next page).

These two sets of statistics must generate a basic conclusion: medical research has failed utterly to come to grips with the problem of cancer. Surgery, radiation and chemotherapy may, in certain individual cases, appear to arrest cancer. However, modern medicine has no essential idea of the cause of cancer. Nor

Chart 2
U.S. Deaths From Cancer, By Site — Per 100,000

	1959	1969	1979
Female Breast cancer	25.51	26.63	26.53
Leukemia — Female	5.72	5.66	5.28
Leukemia — Male	4.78	9.19	8.79
Prostrate	20.34	20.46	22.95
Male Colon-Rectum	25.53	26.01	25.68
Male Pancreas	10.23	11.34	10.90
Female Pancreas	6.20	6.94	7.14
Male — Lung	36.44	56.33	71.14
Female — Lung	5.54	10.47	19.84

Chart 3
Appropriations for the National Cancer Institute
1938 - 1978

1938	$ 400,000
1939	400,000
1947	1,820,900
1948	14,500,000
1949	22,000,000
1957	48,432,000
1958	56,402,000
1959	75,268,000
1967	175,656,000
1968	183,356,000
1969	185,149,500
1970	190,486,063
1971	230,383,000
1972	378,794,000
1973	492,205,000
1974	551,191,500
1975	691,666,000
1976	761,727,000
Transition Quarter	152,901,000
1977	815,000,000
1978	867,136,000

has medicine any concept for prevention and cure of cancer; nor can it seemingly prevent the increase in cancer deaths.

If we believe our establishment media, the United States is the healthiest country in the world. We have the finest trained doctors (no foreign doctor is allowed to practice here without additional training); our nurses have bachelors and even masters degrees; we have superb medical, diagnostic and health care equipment; and our hospitals are the last word in architectural design and efficient treatment of the sick.

These glowing statistics do not tell the whole story. The United States is fast becoming one of the sickest countries in the world and in some diseases, such as cancer, already ranks among the sickest.

It is true that some diseases caused by viruses, so-called pathogenic diseases, have been eliminated and others controlled by medical research. When it comes to diseases of the whole body, the metabolic diseases — which, as we shall show, include cancer — billions of dollars worth of research and equipment have not begun to identify the nature of the solutions.

A basic premise held by most orthodox medical practitioners is that cancer is a local disease, not a metabolic disease. They believe that cancer consists of a lesion, usually in the form of a bump or lump which appears in the breast, on the lung, on the skin, or in some other location in the body. This primary lesion is the result of some activity in the form of an invading virus, or carcinogenic (a cancer-causing irritant) action at the site.

Orthodox treatment, therefore, follows the localized route — usually surgery to remove the offending tumor mass. While early surgeons were content to remove the tumorous mass, it later became evident that cancer cells also invaded adjacent normal tissue. So subsequent surgery included the removal not only of the tumorous mass, but also of a great amount of normal tissue in the adjacent area. In breast surgery, for example, a mastectomy (removal of the breast) removes not only the tumor itself, but also muscle, connective tissue, and lymph glands in the auxilliary area. More recently, surgeons have become more ambitious; to stop a slow-growing tumor, a full quarter of a man was removed. In the most severe cases, a man was actually cut in two, losing both legs, the hips, and all of the external reproductive organs. (See photograph on page 9.)

A second type of localized treatment is to radiate the tumor site with powerful rays known to kill cancer cells. The first objective of radiation is to kill the tumor, and the second is to kill a portion of the adjacent normal tissue into which cancer cells may have infiltrated. The major problem with radiation is that the rays are in no way selective; burn damage, therefore, will occur in normal as well as cancerous tissues. Hair loss also frequently accompanies radiation, due to a disruption of protein metabolism.

A third type of treatment is chemotherapy, designed to selectively kill the cancer cells by taking advantage of their high rate of reproductive activity. Theoretically, chemotherapy should also kill cancer cells circulating in the blood-stream moving to the other areas of the body. In carrying out these functions, however, chemotherapeutic agents are non-selective; they also affect other organ systems of the body with naturally-high cell reproduction. The list of undesirable side effects is long. These side effects differ depending upon the individual and the specific chemotherapeutic agent used, but include loss of hair and reduced ability to assimilate food. Quality of life is all but destroyed and in many cases, death can result from the agent instead of from the disease.

One common factor in all these treatments is that they are unnatural to the human body. They mutilate, burn, or poison. The success rate of these treatments has been anything but spectacular. The basic fallacy in them is that they are harmful to the body which is the host to a malignancy and which should be strengthened, not weakened, against the ravages of this parasitic disease.

Crisis Medicine vs. Preventive Medicine

Most American doctors are dedicated men and women who, along with their own loved ones, are vulnerable to the ravages of

Translumbar amputation (hemicorporectomy), a severe case of orthodox cancer treatment at work.

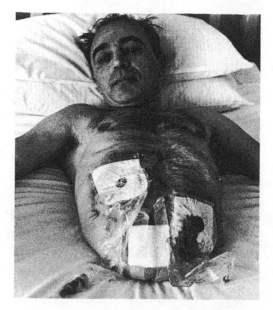

cancer. It would be unrealistic to imply that they are not as individually concerned as all of us in mitigating the suffering caused by this dread disease. No doubt the surgeon wielding his talented scalpel during a mastectomy, the highly trained radiologist burning his target with beams of cobalt, or the well-trained chemotherapist while mixing his poisons, believe they are providing the best care medical science has to offer.

To the extent of the training and knowledge these practitioners have received, this is true. Unfortunately, as you will discover as you read on, the knowledge at their command is supplied by a powerful medical-industrial-governmental axis whose multiple vested interests make total solution of disease financially ruinous and prevention of disease unprofitable.

America has the best equipped and most heavily financed institutions of medical learning in the world. Our medical students are brainwashed into believing that the subsidized education they receive is based upon exacting science. What they are being taught must not be questioned; what they are not taught does not exist. Medical school is not the place for an original thinker and is often the repositiory of entrenched medical error.

Major institutions of medical learning in the U.S. are, without exception, subsidized by the foundations and grants of a multibillion-dollar drug industry. This industry is repaid for its largess with countless prescriptions written by its student proteges. This drug-financed educational program has a post-graduate extension where a myriad of drug company salesmen continue to educate the practicing doctors in the latest drugs and machines available, through them, to their patients.

Thus, we see that it is sound business practice, not philanthropy, that ordains the funneling of drug company profits into education and even directs financial support of the AMA itself, through AMA journal advertising. The result is a medical community that thrives on sickness. The entire financial circle depends upon the continuing flow of high-priced drugs, modalities and procedures to be prescribed when the patient becomes sick.

Notes — CHAPTER ONE

1. American Cancer Society, *Cancer Statistics,* 1979
   Professional Education Publication (New York, 1979).

2. Robert Houston

3. Ibid.

4. *Cancer Statistics.*

5. Ibid.

CHAPTER 2:

Prevention vs. Treatment — the War on Answers

"With superior knowledge the physician cures before the illness is manifested... with inferior knowledge the physician can but attempt to care for the illness he was unable to prevent."

Ancient Chinese proverb

Fortunately, there is a growing body of physicians who believe that the Creator, the greatest healer of all, has designed the human body for wellness, not sickness. If we use a degree of common sense we will find, within our own bodies and the biological environment surrounding us, the preventives against metabolic diseases, as opposed to the crisis medicine of orthodoxy — where treatment commences only when the symptoms appear. In cancer, the symptom is manifested in a lesion, a lump or bump. In this book we will emphasize preventive medicine and how to avoid the symptoms that make us candidates for crisis medicine.

The normal state of the human body is one of health, i.e., an efficient-functioning organic system. It is a steady state, a state of no disease, known to doctors as *homeostasis*.

When this normal state is disturbed in some manner by environment, junk foods, too much smoking and alcohol or other drugs, or by nutrition deficiencies, normal cellular function is altered. One cigarette or one cola drink has little or no effect on the body balance. The cumulative ingestion of cigarettes and junk food on a daily basis is a continuing assault on the body's natural balance that breaks down the system and ultimately leads to metabolic disease. One of these diseases is cancer

Since it is normal for the body to be healthy, it will continually try to maintain that state. If that normalcy is thrown off-balance or out-of-rhythm in any way, the body's own homeostatic mechanisms will try to bring it back. If we get a cold and suffer symptons of a runny nose, slight fever, aching bones, etc., we know that, given enough time, our body will restore itself to health. For some unexplained reason, orthodox medicine draws a line. They say this is fine for some diseases but it is not fine for others. That just is not true! The homeostatic mechanism of the body should be working for *all* diseases.

Suppose an individual stood on a street corner during a freezing-cold winter day, clad only in a bathing suit. The homeostatic mechanism of that person's body would immediately spring into action and he or she would start to shiver. Shivering is a muscular contraction and since muscular contraction produces heat, the heat would be transmitted into the bloodstream. In spite of the fact that it was 30° below zero, body temperature would stay right at 98.6°.

This also applies to nutrition. The body can stand a certain amount of junk food. You can eat marshmallow-filled goodies for breakfast, TV dinners at night, be subjected to all kinds of stress and environmental pollutants, and the body will make adjustments to try to stay healthy. Unfortunately the homeostatic mechanisms in the human body are not infinite — they wear out.

Let us go back to that freezing street corner. Eventually the homeostatic mechanisms that are bringing our shivering subject back to 98.6° are going to be overextended and wear out. Shivering will stop and the inevitable result will be death from exposure. The body can anticipate and handle only so much excess. By the same token, the junk foods, stress and bad environments can be tolerated only so long. Eventually our protective mechanisms will stop and the result is disease. Maintaining homeostasis is very important. The body just cannot take constant overextension of this important mechanism.

At 7:30 in the morning, how many men are driving to work with a cup of coffee and a sweet roll in their hand for breakfast? How many drivers of big 18-wheeler trucks confine their breakfast to coffee and doughnuts after a night of driving?

Fast-order outlets serve a typical lunch of hamburger, French fries and cola. The body just cannot take that kind of punishment. The body seeks a balance. Strategic vitamins and minerals (B1, B3, B6, B12 and chromium) are depleted from the body in an attempt to make up for what cannot be obtained from incomplete foods, and to protect against their harmful ingredients.

Paul Wedel, M.D., himself a recovered cancer patient, was, as a young World War II army lieutenant, put in charge of rehabilitating the victims of one of the largest Nazi concentration camps. His first order to his troops upon reaching the camp was not to give newly rescued inmates any provisions from their own knapsacks. The camp inmates had been living only on water that had been used in cooking cabbage and some carrots. Many of these poor unfortunates were barely alive. Within the first four days many of the U.S. soldiers disobeyed Wedel's order and surreptitiously slipped candy bars to the inmates, thinking they were being merciful. As a direct result of this misplaced kindness approximately 300 inmates died. The last of the vitamins and minerals in their systems were depleted in their bodies' attempt to compensate for the ingestion of this tempting non-food.

In most instances we are better off eating nothing than eating a sugary snack which will actually leach vital vitamins and minerals during the digestive process. Consider some of the manufactured edibles we dignify with the name "food" when they are actually non-foods. There are many artificial foods on the supermarket shelves. In a restaurant, for breakfast, they give you little creamers in white cartons. What do you read on the lid of the carton? 100% non-milk. That tells you what it is not. But now, what *is* it? The ingredients listed are: water, corn syrup, partially hydrogenated soybean oil, mono and diglycerides, sodium caseinate, dipotassium phosphate, sodium stearoyl 2, lactylate, artificial flavor and color (beta carotene). What they are really doing is turning the coffee from a dark color to a lighter color with chemicals made palatable with sugar.

Next time you go to the supermarket take along a pad with you — you will *need* a long one — and write down the names of the chemicals in the prepared foods you customarily purchase.

Take Fig Newtons, for example. Read the label. Regardless of who manufactures it, there is artificial fig flavor added. Now why add artificial fig flavor to something that tastes as good as figs? Because they either pick the figs when they are unripe and have little nutrition or no flavor — or they pick them ripe and the processing is so drastic that it destroys the naturalness of everything. So, flavor is added. And how about brown or white bread? White bread is refined white flour, but brown breads are also made with refined white flour with carmel color added. Or white sugar? Brown sugar is the same thing; it's white sugar, with caramel color added. If you assembled on a plate all the things you had eaten in a week, plus all the chemicals in them, you would not feed it to an animal.

Non-food or junk food is causing an unprecedented increase in the breakdown of the homeostatic mechanism. As soon as that mechanism breaks down the body becomes diseased. Metabolic degenerative diseases used to be diseases of the aged. Not any more. We now have people under 30 with arthritis, arterial sclerosis, heart disease, etc. — all the diseases of the elderly. Which lends credence to the point that it is not time that ages us; it is disease that does this. Old age is not a number, it is a feeling and those with poor health feel it much sooner.

As long as the American people continue to consume junk non-foods and chemicals and remain unwarned by the established medical community, we come to an inevitable conclusion: there is no health care in the United States today. What we have is disease care, or crisis medicine. Doctors are not trained to prevent disease, only to try curing a disease when it occurs.

To quote Andrew McNaughton, head of the McNaughton Foundation and pioneer researcher, "Currently, the emphasis in medicine is more on the treatment of disease than on the maintenance of health. Yet, the emphasis is slowly shifting. As knowledge increases, the pace is quickening.

"It is an open secret that there exists in the U.S.A. for incomprehensible reasons — or rather, very comprehensible ones — considerable opposition against prevention of malignancies with nitriloside therapy."

Dr. Hans A. Nieper in **Krebsgeschehen**
1972/4

The Failure of Establishment Research

That modern medical research — with all its sophisticated techniques and vast investment of money and skills — has failed to resolve the disease of cancer is undeniable. Moreover, the failure was recognized many years ago, over 40 in fact. A book entitled *Cancer: The Failure of Modern Research* was published as far back as 1936.[1] And as we noted in the preceding chapter, cancer mortality rates have risen considerably since the 1930s. By 1925 a medical journal had reported, "Of all the people alive on this globe today more than 100 million are doomed to die from cancer."[2] A year later, in 1926, a British surgeon wrote: "To show how little use medical research has been in this direction, one need only call attention to the fact that, within the last three years, an important research body, confirmed by eminent opinion, stated that food has nothing to do with cancer."[3]

In the 1920s, eminent medical opinion dismissed any possibility that nutrition might be related to cancer. While lack of knowledge on the relationship between nutrition and cancer might be misunderstood in the 1920s, it is remarkable that the relationship is still denied with the advanced nutritional knowledge available to us in the 1980s.

One articulate enemy of the metabolic and nutritional approach to cancer research is Victor Herbert, M.D., Professor of Medicine at the State University of New York, and a speaker at conferences sponsored by the food industry. Dr. Herbert argues, "Inspect any medical school's textbook of medicine or ask your doctor. They will tell you that most diseases have nothing to do with diet."[4] This is *prima facie* evidence, to scientific minds like Dr. Herbert's. What is not in the medical textbooks he has read either does not exist or is not worth considering.

Yet on the other hand, as early as 1915 a book by Frederick L. Hoffman, *The Mortality From Cancer Throughout the World,* discussed the links between nutrition and cancer: "Based upon more general considerations, the opinion has frequently been advanced by ancient and modern writers that there is a direct relationship between diet and cancer frequency, and particularly has this been claimed to be the case in regard to the excessive consumption of salt and meat. The per capita rise in the meat consumption of the principle civilized countries has often been referred to as a causative factor in the corresponding rise in the cancer death rate."[5]

Another early writer, W. R. Williams, in *The Natural History of Cancer,* also reported a link between cancer and diet:

"It may be well to recall the fact that although cancer is remarkably rare in vegetarian communities, complete exemption cannot be claimed for such; and the same is true of herbivorous (plant-eating) communities as compared with carnivorous (meat-eating) groups." Williams is, however, convinced by overwhelming evidence "that the incidence of cancer is largely conditioned by nutrition."[6]

Famed Albert Schweitzer made a related comment, although its significance has been lost on the medical world: "On my arrival in Gabon, in 1913, I was astonished to encounter no cases of cancer. I saw none among the natives two-hundred miles from the coast.

"I cannot, of course, say positively that there was no cancer at all, but, like other frontier doctors, I can only say that if any cases existed they must have been quite rare. This absence of cancer seemed to be due to the difference in nutrition of the natives, as compared to the Europeans."[7]

In more recent times, it is been widely known that people with specific types of diets are remarkably cancer free. For example,

Utah has a lower cancer rate than almost any other area in the United States — only 88.7 deaths from cancer per 100,000, compared to New York with 192 deaths per 100,000. Why? A plausible explanation may be the concentration of Mormons in Utah and the diet followed by the Mormons. There is a doctrine of the Mormon Church: "... a law of health (the 'Word of Wisdom') that counsels against the use of tobacco, alcoholic beverages, tea and coffee, and emphasizes the use of grains, wholesome herbs and fruits for the benefit and health of man."

Another possible factor is the unique research done by Dr. W. Schrauzer on the presence or absence of selenium in the soil. Dr. Schrauzer believes if our soil, and consequently the food grown on that soil, contained adequate selenium, cancer would be reduced by an astounding rate of 75 percent. Much of Utah's soil has a higher than average selenium content.

In brief, we can find observations extending back over a century from numerous sources suggesting some relationship between cancer and diet — certainly enough to suggest that medical research explore the relationship. The failure of modern cancer research is essentially its failure to break out of the, so far, fruitless tunnel-vision search for viral causes of cancer and explore as well the hypothesis of nutritional cause.

In spite of a multimillion-dollar budget — and a mandate from American contributors to explore *every possible avenue* of cancer prevention and control — we are unable to discover in any ACS literature published from 1950 to 1979 where one cent of these millions has been spent on investigating diet and nutrition as a contributory cause of cancer.

The inability or unwillingness of orthodox medicine to develop research along the lines of nutritional deficiencies as the explanation for cancer is not the end of the story of establishment medicine's failure. Where non-medical pressure has pushed the medical establishment into minor research activity on nutrition, the results have been suppressed.

A classic example is the work of Kanematsu Sugiura, M.D., at Memorial Sloan-Kettering Cancer Institute. Some years ago, Dr.

Sugiura was intrigued by the apparent usefulness of amygdalin (a natural substance contained in many edible seeds and plants that have mostly been eliminated from modern man's diet) as a cancer retardant, and instituted some experiments at Sloan-Kettering. Following is a summary conclusion from one of Dr. Sugiura's early experiments which notes "inhibition of growth," "regression" of tumors, and "better health and appearance" in mice under amygdalin treatment:

"Amygdalin in i.p. doses of 1000-2000 mg/kg/day causes significant inhibition of spontaneous mammary tumors in a highly inbred mouse, there is significant inhibition of the formation of lung metastases and it possibly prevents, to an uncertain degree, the formation of new tumors, regardless of the age of the mouse. Greater inhibition of tumor growth was seen in smaller spontaneous tumors of this strain.

"In Swiss Webster albino females with both large and small spontaneous mammary tumors, amygdalin caused regression in 80% of animals studied and complete regression in 40%. The complete regressions occurred only in small tumors on non-inbred mice.

"All treated animals maintained better health and appearance than the controls."[8]

What was the fate of this promising work? Sloan-Kettering announced that the results were not significant and suppressed the report. Fortunately, individuals within Sloan-Kettering had a more sensitive concept of scientific freedom and "leaked" the report to the outside world.

Profitability of Cancer Drugs

Why would establishment medicine suppress and ignore a promising research path? The simplest answer is that there is no profit in nutrition for drug companies, which are locked into an association with orthodox medical research and practice. Why?

A more abstract answer would say it was pride, prejudice and vested interest.

The production and sale of drugs for cancer treatment is a gigantic and profitable business, in contrast to the low profit generated by natural foods and substances. Antineoplastic agents, the narrowest possible definition of those drugs used for cancer control and treatment, account for over $100 million in sales per year. A wider definition of cancer drugs, including anesthetics, hormonal preparations affecting neoplasms and other cancer-related drugs, puts the cancer drug industry in the $1 billion-a-year category.

These cancer treatment drugs are produced by a dozen or so major pharmaceutical firms whose annual financial statements confirm that this is a highly profitable business. Eli Lilly is 42nd in profitability among all U.S. firms and generates a 23 percent return on equity for its owners. Upjohn is 154th in profitability among U.S. companies and yields a 17 percent return on equity for its owners.

When we look in detail at the anti-cancer drugs produced and sold by these and other drug companies, it is extraordinary that their products receive FDA approval as being safe for human use. The toxic effects of anti-cancer drugs bring to mind a statement once made by Dr. Ernst Krebs, Jr.:

> "Chemotherapy and radiation will make the ancient method of drilling holes in a patient's head to permit escape of demons to cure madness look relatively advanced... toxic chemotherapy is a hoax. It is premeditated murder. Use of cobalt and other methods of cancer treatment popular today closes the door on cure."[9]

The cost to the patient of the orthodox cancer "treatment" is horrendous. The 1973 preinflation figure from the ACS factbook puts it between $19,000 and $50,000. The average price tag is about $30,000 for medical services alone, except in minor cases such as skin cancer. Hospital costs run about $200 per day, so an average hospital stay of 15 days adds up to several thousand dollars. The total loss of income in the U.S. from cancer probably runs $30 billion a year.

Anti-Cancer Drugs: Toxic and Useless

Proponents of orthodox chemotherapeutic treatment for cancer continually allude to purported toxic reactions caused by the natural foods we will recommend in this book which are used in the dietary approach to cancer control. Included in their unsupported list of dangerous items are such natural foods as amygdalin, vitamin A, and enzymes from the lentil bean, all of which are totally nontoxic when taken in appropriate amounts.

Chart 4 lists some of the well-known and widely prescribed anti-cancer drugs used by orthodox medical practitioners. Manufacturers, brand names, efficacy and toxicity are as recorded in orthodoxy's own *Physician's Desk Reference*.[10]

Two observations can be made about the anti-cancer drugs listed in Chart 4 (page 21):

1. These "anti-cancer" drugs are less than efficacious and, in many cases, not curative at all.

2. These drugs are always highly toxic, sometimes fatally so, yet they receive FDA approval as "safe" drugs.

More-detailed extracts on a few selected drugs from the *Physician's Desk Reference* suggest the extremely limited value and highly dangerous side effects produced:

Leukeran

The aklylating agent Leukeran (chlorambucil) is a derivative of nitrogen mustard, under U.S. Patent No. 2,944,079, manufactured by Burroughs Wellcome Co. It is described as a "potent" drug used in treatment of leukemia. It is not curative but produces "striking remissions" and is used with warnings: "Excessive or prolonged dosage will produce severe bone marrow depression. Severe neutropenia (abnormally small numbers of neutrophils in the circulating blood) is related to dosage in a significant number of cases and there is a real risk of causing irreversible bone marrow damage."

Leukeran has FDA approval as a safe drug.

Chart 4
DRUGS USED FOR CANCER
(according to the National Cancer Institute)

GENERIC NAME	BRAND NAME	MANUFACTURER	EFFICACY, according to Physicians Desk Reference	TOXICITY
BUSULFAN (sulfonic ester, alkylating agent)	"MYLERAN"	Burroughs, Wellcome	"Of value, not curative"	"Toxic effects"
CHLORAMBUCIL (alkylating agent)	"LEUKERAN"	Burroughs, Wellcome	"not curative but produces remissions"	"a potent drug... patients must be followed carefully to avoid irreversible damage to the bone marrow"
CYTOXAN (Cyclophosphamide)	"CYTOXAN"	Mead, Johnson	"interferes with growth of cancer (and normal cells). Has orcogenic (cancer creating) possibilities"	Numerous adverse reactions including "severe, even fatal" reactions
PIPOBROMAN	"VERCYTE"	Abbott	Mechanism not known, "useful"	"Adverse reactions reported: nausea, vomiting, cramping, diarrhea, skin rash"
TRIETHYLENETHIO-PHOSPHORAMIDE	"THIOTEPA"	Lederle	Widely used with "varying results"	Complications can cause death unless checked promptly
CYTARABINE	"CYTOSAR"	Upjohn	"Few with solid tumors have benefited from the drug"	Highly toxic and numerous reactions
5-FLUOROURACIL	"5-FU"	Roche	"Effective in palliative management of some cancers... not for patients in poor nutritional state."	Possibility of "severe toxic reactions"
MERCAPTOPURINE	"PURINETHOL"	Burroughs, Wellcome	Believed to interfere with nucleic acid biosynthesis	Severe toxic reactions with no known antagonist.
METHOTREXATE		Lederle	Inhibits growth of cell tissue	Highly toxic, deaths have been reported
THIOGUANINE		Burroughs, Wellcome	Not effective against solid tumors	Toxic, no know antagonist.
VINBLASTINE SULFATE	"VELBAN"	Eli Lilly	Relieves pain, has produced temporary reduction in tumors	Some adverse reactions
VINCRISTINE SULFATE	"ONCOVIN"	Eli Lilly	Indicated in acute leukemia	Adverse reactions are reversible but overdose can have fatal outcome.

Cytoxan

Cytoxan (cyclophosphamide) is a synthethic drug related to the nitrogen mustards, classified as one of the anti-cancer alkylating agents, and manufactured by Mead Johnson and Company. It interferes with the growth of cancer "and, to some extent, certain normal tissues." Among warnings for use is the disclosure that "Cytoxan has been reported to have oncogenic activity in rats and mice," i.e., it can cause cancer. It is recommended that "the possibility that it may have oncogenic potential in humans should be considered." The adverse reactions for Cytoxan are numerous. Leukopenia is an "expected effect." Nausea and vomiting are common. Sterile hemorrhagic cystitis can result from Cytoxan **"this can be severe, even fatal, and is probably due to metabolites in the urine.** Other complications can occur."

Cytoxan has FDA approval as a safe drug.

Vercyte

Vercyte (pipobroman) is another aklylating agent, manufactured by Abbott Laboratories. According to the *Physician's Desk Reference,* "The mechanism of action is unknown and the metabolic fate and route of excretion are unknown." However it is known that Vercyte frequently causes "bone marrow depression." It is not recommended for use in children under age 15 "because no significant clinical effect has been shown with patients in this age group."

Vercyte has FDA approval as a safe drug.

Thiotepa

Thiotepa is an aklylating agent used in conventional treatment of cancer, and manufacturered by Lederle Laboratories. It is used "with varying results" in a wide variety of neoplasms. It is "highly toxic," can create serious complications which "unless checked promptly... may lead to death." There is no known antidote for an overdose of Thiotepa and numerous adverse reactions include local pain, nausea, dizziness, headache.

Thiotepa has FDA approval as a safe drug.

Cytosar

Cytosar was synthesized simultaneously by University of California Laboratories and the Upjohn Company. The results in the first 389 cases used are summarized in Chart 5. Almost 60 percent indicated no beneficial response and only 6.7 percent of cases had "complete remission." On the other hand, there are major known toxic effects and an extremely high percentage of patients report adverse reactions. Experimental studies indicated that some transplanted mouse tumors were inhibited, but there is no activity against rat tumors. Further studies show that Cytosar is immunosuppressive, i.e., it suppresses the body's natural immunological responses and is a potent bone marrow depressant. Other effects reported were:

Leukopenia 65.9 percent

Bone Marrow Suppression 19.4 percent

Nausea 15.6 percent

Vomiting 14.2 percent

"Given large doses, patients are frequently nauseated and may vomit for several hours post injection."

Cytosar has FDA approval as a safe drug.

Chart 5
Results of Tests with Cytosar (First 389 Cases)

Total Number Patients Treated	Complete Remission	Partial Remission	Improved	No Beneficial Response	Inadequate Trial
235 adults (acute leukemia)	19	30	22	137	27
154 children (Leukemia)	7	40	9	89	9
TOTALS					
389	26	70	31	226	36
100 per cent	6.7%	18.0%	8.0%	58.1%	9.2%

5-Fluorouracil

The antimetaboite 5-FU is manufactured under the brand name of Hoffman-La Roche Laboratories, and is used as a palliative in some cancers that cannot be treated surgically. 5-FU is very toxic and has to be used with extreme caution, treatment being discontinued if any one of several adverse indications appear. It is described as a "highly toxic drug with a narrow margin of safety." Fatalities may be encountered even in patients in relatively good condition. It is so dangerous that it is recommended that therapy be discontinued at the end of the 12th day even if no toxicity has become apparent.

Its efficacy is rather questionable: the effect may be to "create a thyamine deficiency which provokes unbalanced growth and death of the cell."

5-Fluorouracil has FDA approval as a safe drug.

Mercaptopurine

Manufactured by Burroughs, Wellcome Co. under the brand name Purinethol. Mercaptopurine is a potent drug used in treatment of acute leukemia. The drug is toxic and effects may be delayed even with highly lethal dosages. Numerous adverse reactions have been recorded and there is no known drug which will counter Mercaptopurine.

Mercaptopurine has FDA approval as a safe drug.

Methotrexate

Methotrexate, manufactured by Lederle Laboratories, is a highly toxic antimetabolite with the possibility of fatal toxic reactions. Deaths have been reported. The action is, supposedly, to prevent growth of malignant tissues without irreversible damage to normal tissue, and it has been used as a palliative in leukemia.

Methotrexate has FDA approval as a safe drug.

Readers are reminded that the foregoing statements of toxicity on FDA-approved drugs are not our editiorial opinion, but are taken directly from the *Physician's Desk Reference,* a volume used to guide the practicing physician in his choice of medication.

Throughout the balance of this book we will advocate the cancer-preventive properties of natural vitamins, including B17 or amygdalin.

Many of the advocates and users of the previously listed dangerous chemicals have the temerity to tell their patients that vitamins and amygdalin are toxic and should, therefore, be avoided. They choose to ignore even the FDA's recent admission that amygdalin is "harmless to both man and beast when used as an essential part of the metabolic approach to cancer."[11]

Although laetrile (vitamin B17 or amygdalin) is not listed in the *Physician's Desk Reference,* the following reactions have been reported by physicians using the pure, natural form of amygdalin, based on clinical human use: temporary lowering of blood pressure, pain reduction, complete pain elimination, increased appetite, weight gain, increased mental acuity, increased energy, subjective remission, objective remission, total remission.

Notes: CHAPTER TWO

1. M. Beddow Bayle, *Cancer: The Failure of Modern Research,* London, 1936.
2. *Surgery, Gynecology and Obstetrics,* 1925.
3. Quoted from *Sunday Express,* London, England, December 27, 1931.
4. Victor Herbert, *The Health Robbers.*
5. F. Hoffman, *The Mortality From Cancer Throughout the World,* 1915.
6. W. R. Williams, *The Natural History of Cancer,* 1927.
7. Alexander Bergulas, *Cancer Nature, Cause and Cure,* Institute Pasteur, Paris, 1935.
8. Kanematsu Sugiura, "A Summary of the Effect of Amygdalin Upon Spontaneous Tumors in Mice." Extracted from confidential Sloan-Kettering report suppressed but "leaked" by staff members.
9. E. T. Krebs, Speech to National Health Federation, Los Angeles, California, 1979.
10. *Physician's Desk Reference*, pp. 671-2.
11. Moertel, NCI Report on Non-Toxicity of Amygdalin.

CHAPTER 3:

What Is Cancer?

"There is a growing awareness among the American people that orthodox medicine is not working because the solutions lie outside the accepted patterns of thought."

Marilyn Ferguson

In recent years, a new and non-orthodox school of thought has emerged which looks upon cancer as a metabolic disease that can be prevented. This new wave of medical practitioners has proven, to its own satisfaction, that cancer is a nutritional deficiency. This nonorthodox school is in violent, daily opposition to the orthodox medical establishment in a battle that rages in the newspapers, in courts and in doctors' offices.

The use of enzymes, vitamins and minerals in the prevention of cancer has generated such organizations as the International Association of Cancer Victims and Friends, the National Health Federation, the Coalition for Alternative Therapy, and the Cancer Control Society. The opponents of the preventive, nutritional approach include the American Medical Association, the U.S. Food and Drug Administration, the American Cancer Society, the Memorial Sloan-Kettering Institute and the National Cancer Institute.

The battle reflects an underlying basic difference in the interpretation of the nature of cancer. Orthodox establishment medicine is straightforward in acknowledging that it does not know the nature of the disease and, therefore, has had only limited success in treatment; at the same time, its approach does reflect an underlying assumption that each type of cancer is a biologically distinctive phenomenon, i.e., that all cancers are different. There are many types of cancer cells and, therefore, many varying explanations and treatments of the phenomenon.

By contrast, the proponents of the metabolic approach embrace various internal change concepts predicated on the fact that a cancer cell is an aberration of a naturally-occurring cell — one that exists in the body as a natural part of the life cycle, but which has malfunctioned and is not being controlled by normal body defenses. This latter position is referred to as the unitarian thesis of cancer.

The orthodox interpretation and the challenging unitarian thesis are irreconcilable, one with the other; either cancer is unitary or it is non-unitarian. In the words of some of the pioneers of the unitarian concept: "... the unitarian thesis holds that the malignant component in all exhibitions of cancer is the same; that this component is not spontaneously created but represents the most primitive cell in the life cycle, the trophoblast cell, gone awry."

The only key program funded by establishment sources that is involved with nutrition as it affects cancer is the Diet, Nutrition and Cancer Program (DNCP) of the National Cancer Institute. This program is only lightly funded, however, and has but a few faltering projects underway. While a river of gold provided by your taxes has been pumped into a mammoth cancer establishment which has failed to produce results, the believers in metabolic medicine have gone ahead without government money. The results of their metabolic nutritional investigation and research are so overwhelmingly positive that the second half of this book is dedicated to offering you a "cookbook" for a healthy life, a dietary guide to healthy living — one in which cancer cannot exist.

In Your Interest or Their Interest?

Cancer research and treatment is riddled with actual and potential conflicts of interest, thus a situation has been created in which there is no incentive to explore new avenues of research, and the financial advantage is to maintain a status quo — an inertial languor that kills 400,000 Americans annually.

The boards of directors of firms producing drugs used in chemotherapy are sprinkled with academics and researchers supposedly involved in the unbiased search for a cancer cure. The most prominent example is Lewis Thomas, president of Memorial Sloan-Kettering Cancer Center, who is also a director of Squibb Corporation, a producer of drugs used in chemotherapy. Other medical people serving as directors of Squibb include Helen M. Ranney, M.D., chairman, Department of Medicine, University of California, San Diego.

Some of the drugs marketed by Squibb and used in cancer treatment and research are:

- Hydroxyurea (Hydrea) used in treatment of chronic leukemia and melanoma.
- Teslac, a hormonal agent used in treatment of breast cancer.

Looking at other drug firms: At the Upjohn Company we find, among its board members, William N. Hubbard, Jr., M.D., and Donald F. Hornig, Ph.D., president of Brown University.

Upjohn produces the following cancer treatment drugs:

- Cytosine Arabinoside used in treatment of leukemia.
- Cortisone used in treatment of leukemia and breast cancer.
- Calusterone used in treatment of breast cancer.
- Halotestin used in treatment of breast cancer.

The Merck & Company, Inc. board of directors includes two prominent medical researcher administrators: Jacques Genest, M.D., director of the Clinical Research Institute of Montreal, and Glenn S. Pound, Ph.D., Dean of Agricultural and Life Sciences, University of Wisconsin. Merck produces alkylating agents used in treatment of breast cancer, melanoma, ovarian and other cancerous disorders.

The Abbott Laboratories' board of directors includes: E. M. Papper, M.D., Dean, School of Medicine, University of Miami, and Boone Powell, M.D., Director, Baylor University Medical Center. Abbott makes Pipobroman used in treatment of leukemia.

In brief, supposedly unbiased cancer researchers have an unhealthy link to and pecuniary interest in the cancer drug-producing companies. If only subconsciously, they cannot dismiss the devastating financial effect a nutritional solution to cancer will have on the drug industry.

The Rockefeller Family Interest in Cancer

The link between production and sale of toxic, useless drugs for cancer treatment and the medical establishment is nowhere more clear than in the case of the Rockefeller family. The family has pecuniary interests in drug production and, at the same time, trusteeship in cancer research and hospital facilities.

In 1949, the late Nelson Rockefeller became a member of the board of the Memorial Sloan-Kettering Institute for Cancer Research and later was named chairman of the board. In light of the Sloan-Kettering suppression of Sugiura's report on amygdalin noted in the preceding chapter, it is interesting that Rockefeller commented as follows on communicating the results of research to others, "... we work very hard at doing this at Memorial and in addition try to get our findings very quickly into the educational system through close relationships with Rockefeller University and Cornell Medical School."

Rockefeller also claimed to have tried to increase federal participation in the fight against cancer, and served six years on the National Cancer Advisory Board.

This powerful, aristocratic family has a significant influence on cancer research. In 1976 the Rockefeller Brothers Fund contributed $2.5 million toward the building program at Memorial Sloan-Kettering Cancer Center, the key U.S. cancer research complex. Lawrence Rockefeller is today chairman of Sloan-Kettering. During U.S. Senate hearings on the nomination of Vice President Nelson Rockefeller, it was revealed that the Rockefeller Brothers Fund was heavily invested in Merck & Co. (manufacturers of the cancer drug Mithracin), Pfizer, Inc.

(manufacturers of antibiotics used in cancer treatments) and Squibb Corporation (manufacturer of the cancer drug Hydrea).

More importantly, the Rockefeller family interests have close interlocks with drug companies. These interlocks were summarized in the Congressional report on the nomination of Nelson Rockefeller for Vice President as follows:

- Ralston Purina, manufacturers of lab chow to feed testing mice: Two interlocks with the Rockefeller family.

- Colgate Palmolive (subsidiary is Kendall). Eighteen percent of its earnings come from surgical products: Four interlocks with the Rockefeller family.

- Bristol Myers: Two interlocks with the Rockefeller family through Bristol Labs and Mead Johnson, manufacturers of BiCNV, CeeNu and Blenoxane.

- Warner Lambert: Two interlocks with the Rockefeller family (through Parke Davis and Warner Chilcott Labs).

- Eli Lilly: Two interlocks with the Rockefeller family; manufacturers Velban, Drolban and Oncovin.

More Profit in Looking For A Cure
Than Finding A Cure

Let us suppose the metabolic-nutritional approach to cancer prevention were to become widespread, and not restricted to those estimated 50,000 Americans willing to risk harassment by bureaucrats and medical associates. What would be the results?

Certainly the size and commercial influence of the lucrative cancer research industry would be drastically reduced. The American Cancer Society, the numerous academics who serve on cancer research boards, the fund raisers and the public relations people would be looking for other work. Manufacturers of radiation equipment, X-ray machines and cobalt machines would suffer drastic cuts in production and revenue. Most alarming (for the drug firms), a whole range of dangerous toxic drugs would no longer be required. A multibillion-dollar industry would be devastated.

To compound the prejudicial problems of these already heavily-vested interests, it now costs between $14 million and $26 million to get a new drug approved by the FDA (1973 pre-inflationary figures). Amygdalin and other natural substances are in the public domain and cannot be patented. No one will invest that large a sum in any substance which cannot be patented, faced with the realization they cannot retrieve their investment.

Thus, the FDA acts as little more than a protective entity in a racket benefiting those drug companies that can well afford these huge sums.

In brief, there is more profit in merely *looking* for a cure for cancer than in actually finding a cure.

CHAPTER 4:

Nutrition:
The New Direction

"If a patient dies of cancer without being informed that there are alternative treatment methods to those of established medical opinion, I believe it would be appropriate for his survivors to sue the doctors who failed to inform him."

Robert C. Atkins, M.D., **Nutrition Breakthrough**

As nutritional knowledge has become more advanced, a small but vocal group of enlightened physicians has concluded, empirically and logically, that cancer is a dietary deficiency disease; it involves, as they see it, specific deficiencies at the cellular level of pancreatic enzymes and deficiencies of amygdalin (vitamin B17), along with associated A, E, C and other vitamin and mineral deficiencies. The logic of this position is supported by the incontestable fact that, without exception, the resolution of all chronic metabolic diseases, when finally discovered, was effected by supplying a missing food factor in the same molecular form as available in nature. There is no logical reason to believe cancer is an exception.

Scurvy: Cured by Vitamin C

Several centuries ago, scurvy — a disease characterized by weakness and hemorrhaging of tissues and pain-racked joints —was a common, often fatal disease among sailors, explorers, and the inhabitants of communities lacking fresh food. So many artificially-fed infants developed scurvy that the dread disease once known as the "sailor's calamity" also became known as the "baby's calamity."

While scurvy today is relatively rare, for the period before 1700 it was a disease capable of causing widespread epidemics, sometimes of catastrophic proportions. People of all walks of life in many nations were once in the painful, raging throes of terminal scurvy. In 1498, Vasco da Gama sailed around the Cape of Good Hope in South Africa. Out of his crew of 160, fully one-quarter succumbed to scurvy.

About the end of the 16th Century it was randomly observed that fresh fruit and vegetables had immediate curative effects on scurvy. In 1593, Sir Richard Hawkins noted and later published, in observations on his voyage into the South Seas, references that natives of the area used sour oranges and lemons as a cure for scurvy, and a similar result was noted among his crew. Yet, for nearly two centuries European doctors refused to consider this simple treatment, used so effectively on island savages and Hawkins' crew; instead, they continued to search the dark, dank hulls of ships for some strange, still undiscovered, source of the disease.

Finally, in 1754, Dr. James Lind, surgeon at the Royal Naval Hospital, Haslar, England, wrote *Treatise on the Scurvy,* in which he described experiments upon sailors and the use of oranges and lemons with both preventive and curative effects. It still took 50 more years for British physicians to finally accept the nutritional control of scurvy and recommend that lime juice be included in sea rations.

Lind's perceptive observations can be applied to present day treatment of cancer. It was observed then that some persons cannot be brought to believe that a disease so fatal and dreadful as scurvy can be prevented or cured by such easy means. They would have more faith in some elaborate composition dignified by the chemical name of an antiscorbutic or similar term of Greek or Latin derivation. Facts are sufficient to convince the unprejudiced; however it is no easy matter to rule out all the prejudices and overturn opinions firmly entrenched by time, custom and the endorsement of respected authorities.

The practical effects of fresh fruit on scurvy were known before there was any understanding of the reason for the effects. And for two centuries ships carried oranges, lemons or vegetables as a preventive against scurvy without understanding the principle of vitamins. In 1804, regulations were introduced into the British Navy requiring use of lime juice in the absence of fresh fruits. This measure was eventually enacted into law by the British Board of Trade in 1865, with the effect of almost eliminating scurvy.

While the empirical cure for scurvy was known, it was not until the early part of the 20th Century that vitamin C was singled out as the specific anti-scurvy element at work. Then followed experiments isolating vitamin C and confirming that a deficiency in it was indeed the cause of scurvy. In sum, it took two centuries to translate empirical observation into action and more than another century before the curative element for scurvy was identified as vitamin C!

Beriberi: Cured by Vitamin B1 (Thiamine)

For thousands of years, beriberi was a major disease in the Far East and various other areas with high consumption of polished rice. In 1882, a Japanese Navy doctor, Takaki, empirically determined beriberi to be a dietary deficiency. There were major problems with food given to Japanese sailors, which in the Japanese Navy consisted largely of polished rice. On one naval voyage there were 169 cases of beriberi out of a total crew of 376, of which no fewer than 25 died. On the next training ship voyage, Takaki substituted a high-protein diet, accidently containing sufficient vitamin B1 to eliminate beriberi. In 1878, 1485 cases of beriberi were reported in the Japanese Navy; by 1888, it was completely eliminated. Similar results were reported from the Dutch East Indies, the Philippines and even inside the United States. It was found by Eijkman in 1897 that beriberi could be induced by feeding polished rice to chickens, and by Funk in 1911 that pigeons could be cured of beriberi by feeding them rice polishings (i.e., the part removed in rice processing).

In 1927, vitamin B was isolated by two Dutch researchers, Jansen and Dunath, and in 1936, vitamin B1 was synthesized. As in the case of vitamin C, we find that the cure for beriberi was determined empirically and then the substance was isolated and synthesized in the laboratory, but not until many years had passed.

Chart 6
Vitamin Deficiency Diseases and Their Cures

Disease	Empirical observation of "cures" for the disease	Testing and hypothesizing	Generally accepted as a vitamin deficiency disease
Scurvy	During 16th and 17th centuries	British Navy in late 18th century. Holst & Frolich (1907-1912)	Early to mid-19th century
Beri-Beri	Takaki in 1877	Tested in Japanese Navy 1886; Suzuki, Funk, Jansen & Donath (1912-1926)	Early 20th century
Rickets	Guenn (1838) to Dibbelt (1909) (concentrating on calcium in diet)	Testing of cod liver oil at London Zoo. Later experiments with rats in U.S.	Early 1922 with separation of Vitamin A into A and D
Pellagra	Goldberger in U.S. noted relationship of pellagra to diet	Voegtlin (1920) Goldberger (1927)	Early 1930's Vitamin B₃ accepted anti-pellagra component.

Pellagra: Cured by Vitamin B3 (Niacin)

As recently as 50 years ago, pellagra was a common disease in the southern part of the United States. In 1917, for example, there were more than 170,000 cases in the southern states, and in South Carolina pellagra ranked second as a cause of death. In 1920, it was found that a diet rich in vitamin B-complex would cure pellagra. In 1927, Dr. J. Goldberger identified the differences between pellagra and beriberi, and determined that vitamin B-complex was pellagra's cure. This eminent medical scholar was ignored by the medical establishment, which was concentrating its research on finding a viral cause of the disease — even though Dr. Goldberger's clinical studies proved conclusively that the disease was concentrated in the southern United States, where the diet of Negroes and poor whites was heavy in maize meal, molasses and meat, which contain insufficient vitamin B3 to prevent pellagra.

Is Cancer A Dietary Deficiency?

Most research programs start with random empirical observations by a researcher looking for a solution to a problem. These seemingly casual observations link a postulated cause to an observed effect and form a preliminary pattern in the mind of the investigator. It is this preliminary pattern which gives rise to the process of hypothesizing, or outlining possible explanations.

In the assault on scurvy, beriberi and pellagra, this cycle of empirical observation — development of explanatory patterns, derivation of and testing of hypotheses — is seen clearly.

In cancer today, establishment science admittedly knows of no general cause for the lump or bump it calls cancer. The establishment "cure" for cancer is to remove the lump or bump by surgery, radiation, or chemical means. Orthodox medicine cannot guarantee that cancer will not recur, nor can it regulate cancer once it has grown beyond a certain point.

On the other hand, for the past century there have been numerous random observations linking cancer to nutrition, paralleling the observations made in the 16th-18th Centuries linking cure of scurvy to fresh fruits and vegetables and the cure of rickets to sunshine and (as later determined) a vitamin D deficiency; and the cure of beriberi was identified to be nutritional during this era, long before vitamin B was isolated and synthesized. These preliminary patterns of observation of action-and-effect developed into the science of hypothesizing and, ultimately, understanding and curing these previously-deadly metabolic diseases.

How extensive then are the empirical observations linking cancer to nutrition? Why has modern research ignored nutrition as a factor in cancer? More than 60 years ago, medical journals reported significant results from controlled experiments on the relationship between diet and cancer. Several researchers confirmed this important relationship that cried out for further investigation. The research was continued by individuals such as biochemist Krebs, but Krebs' work has been arbitrarily rejected by modern medicine.

In 1911, Peyton Rous reported in the *Proceedings of the Society for Experimental Biology and Medicine:* "Experimental work shows that the development of tumor grafts can in many cases be prevented or retarded by underfeeding the host or by putting it on a special diet." Further work along these lines was reported by Rous in the *Journal of Experimental Medicine.*

Then, in 1913, a group of three researchers reported similar findings in the *Journal of Biological Chemistry,* and cited the unfavorable influence of poor nutrition on tumor growth. In this article, authors Sweet, Corson-White and Saxon refer to other researchers who had noted in their studies the effects of feeding rats with combinations of pure vegetable protein and a number of diets that completely retarded the normal growth of the animals. These findings concluded that susceptibility to transplantable tumors can be influenced positively or negatively by diet.

This early experimental evidence, under controlled conditions, has been totally ignored by establishment medicine and government reporters. For example, Michael B. Shimkin in *Science and Cancer,* the official booklet put out by the U.S. Department of Health, Education and Welfare, claims: "There is no diet that prevents cancer in man. Treatment of cancer by diet alone is in the realm of quackery." In science one cannot prove a negative statement, but Shimkin's statement also introduces another peculiarity of establishment medicine, i.e., its habit of dismissing opponents and critics as "quacks". We shall see later that, if we apply the same "quackery" criteria to orthodox medicine, the "quacks" are none other than establishment researchers themselves, and institutions pretending to have a cure they neither have nor can find.

In any event, this must be the first time that experimental work reported in the *Journal of Biological Chemistry* and the *Journal of Experimental Medicine* has been dismissed as "quackery".

With the exception of the suppressed Sloan-Kettering experiment, modern research is notable in its lack of interest in the nutritional approach. Yet, establishment medicine is well aware of scientific criteria and quote them at length when they appear to be to its own benefit when attacking the use of nutritional and ancillary therapy.

Furthermore, there is a scientific axiom, fundamental to scientific research, to the effect that a negative proposition cannot be proven. In other words, it is unscientific to make the statement "there is no diet that prevents cancer in man." This is a negative statement unsupported by scientific proof. It makes Dr. Shimkin the "quack" and places the Department of Health, Education and Welfare itself in a position of publishing unscientific claims and supporting "quackery". Only by overcoming the prejudicial quackery of consensus medicine have pernicious anemia, beriberi, rickets, pellagra, goiter and a host of other metabolic diseases been conquered. In every case the cause was nutritional deficiency and the cure was in the reversal of that deficiency. The final resolution of cancer will likewise be found in nutrition.

The Geography of Cancer

The monumental failure by establishment medicine to come to grips with cancer suggests that somewhere along the line, over the past century, medical research has taken a wrong turn. The recent response in Washington has been to throw money, and more money, at the problem — particularly under Nixon's National Cancer Attack Act of 1971. This approach may make good politics but it makes bad cancer research. If the basic approach is in error, then the investment of more funds will compound, rather than solve, the cancer problem. (Good money thrown after bad!)

The common-sense approach, for both scientists and laymen, is to step back and take a fresh look at cancer. If the rate of cancer deaths has been increasing over the past century and at an accelerated rate in this current decade (all this acceleration occurring while waging a massive research attack), then we have to logically assume:

(a) that present treatments are, in effect, no cure; and,

(b) that some pervasive causative factor is at work, is multiplying, and that establishment research has no awareness of its nature or its workings.

The medical establishment maintains a monopoly on medical research; it refuses to allow, or even test, what it calls "unproven methods." In brief, there is a monopoly of thinking in medical research which inhibits new directions. The shrill attacks on "unproven methods," and, in the U.S., use of the police power of the state to forcibly prevent and imprison any doctor or researcher who attempts to probe "unproven methods," is a distinct sign of uncertainty — i.e., the establishment's inability to find a solution within its *own* framework of analysis and past knowledge.

The very vehemence of the attacks by orthodox medicine on therapies not originated by the establishment is not only a rejection of free choice of therapy but a sign of self-admitted failure.

This bias for well-worn established research paths was explained to a congressional committee by Clinton R. Miller of the National Health Federation in 1971:

"You see, bias can occur in very honest and sincere people. I have never met an unbiased person in my life and I hope I never do. I think it is a myth that we have bought that scientists are less biased than politicians or than people with strong religious convictions.

"We have assumed, and have actually been taught, that there is something in science that removes bias, and this simply is not so." (That today's medical science is still biased against vitamin and nutritional research, there can be no doubt.) "The American cancer establishment," Miller continued, "has looked only at highly toxic chemotherapeutic agents that they have tried at the National Cancer Institute."

"The minute that an agent gets to the gentleness of a natural food or vitamin they will not even try it. What is more important, they will not allow it to be tried on others."

Let us develop the implications of Clinton Miller's arguments. Let us assume a tire blows on your car. You do not have to be a tire manufacturer to know that the tire is no longer functioning. You identify the problem — that is, make an initial hypothesis that the tire has blown — and take the car at once to a garage. You do not continue driving. You do not normally try to fix it yourself. You identify the problem and adopt the required solution.

Now suppose all four tires blow at the same time. One does not have to be a tire manufacturer to take simple actions and make deductions. If all tires were bought at the same time from the same manufacturer and blow under the same conditions, then one is justified in calling attention to the manufacturer of a probable defect in his tire manufacturing methods. Again, we identify a problem and take first steps, when the indicators suggest a direction calling for research to solve the problem.

Similarly, one does not have to be a medical researcher to identify the logical direction in cancer or to identify bias. We cannot undertake the research ourselves, but we can make initial observations and draw initial conclusions. Let us make one such simple observation: the incidence of cancer in Utah is far lower than the incidence of cancer in the rest of the United States — a simple, irrefutable observation. Why? Again, intelligent laymen will ask what is different about Utah from the rest of the U.S.? A preliminary answer might be the significant influence of the Church of Latter-Day Saints.

The low incidence of cancer in Utah has not gone unnoticed. The Utah division of the American Cancer Society published a report on the phenomenon. The report states there was an assumption, at first, that the difference between Utah and the rest of the U.S. was attributable to a difference in the age levels of statistical study groups. This, however, proved to be erroneous. The disparity, after adjusting for age differentials, narrowed somewhat; but this does not, according to the ACS report, "sufficiently explain Utah's lower rates." The Utah data was compared with data for the State of Connecticut, which maintains a Tumor Registry. The evidence, it was concluded, "indicates that Utah has an unusual pattern of both new cases of cancer and mortality from cancer. The determinants of this are not clear to the American Cancer Society. Certainly a reduced amount of cigarette consumption in the population is one factor. However, this does not fully explain differences present in such sites as colon, rectum, etc." The report adds that Utah should "begin detailed research projects" to define the areas of difference and "explore determinants of these differences." Then follows a series of detailed statistical analyses of Utah cancer by anatomical location — acute leukemia, cancer of the stomach, colon, etc. Most noticeably, the report does not attempt to acknowledge —or even hint at — any significance in the fact that dietary differences between Utah and Connecticut seem to indicate there are fruitful paths for further research. Logic would suggest that, given the data offered in the report, a researcher should explore for EXOGENOUS (outside the body) factors. But alas, the report distinguishes tumors only by site location *in the body* and makes no attempt to explore the premise that factors of an external origin could be responsible.

From the viewpoint of methodology, it is extraordinary that the American Cancer Society writers come to grips with the Utah phenomenon only within the philosophical framework of traditional, narrow-minded establishment reasoning. These writers —as though their eyes were covered with horse blinders — attribute and allocate tumors to various parts of the body. Never mind the correct methodological procedure, which is to first list all the possible differences between Utah and other geographical areas of the United States, then arrive at the ultimate explanations by a process of deduction based on experimentation.

By contrast, the first and only step of this ACS report is to divide cancers into body sites and arrive at the momentous conclusion that in Utah some type of neoplasms are more common that others. In recommending further work, the report suggests that "The Utah Tumor Registry should now begin detailed research projects to further define the areas of major differences between the U.S. and other selective populations and explore determinants of these differences."

Apart from a casual reference to cigarette smoking, no attempt is made to step back from the Utah data and look at it in the broadest possible context. The methodological defect is a research approach that counts trees very effectively but ignores the forest as a whole — and this is the fatal reason why establishment research has so utterly failed to solve the cancer epidemic. It confirms the validity of Clinton Miller's charge of bias.

While no areas of the U.S. are completely cancer-free, some states have a significantly low incidence of cancer which, as in Utah, cannot be explained by either statistical errors or establishment practice.

Quite obviously, these statistics require explanation, since no valid explanation exists in establishment medical doctrine. However, one simple plausible explanation stands out a mile: some common environmental factor — perhaps diet or nutrition — has a geographical variation, and this variation may be responsible, in turn, for varying cancer death rates. This explanation, when we consider the Mormon diet in Utah, becomes more plausible —overwhelmingly so when we look at other instances of relationships between cancer and diet.

It has long been recognized that Seventh-Day Adventists have lower cancer incidence than the general population. This is a widely-dispersed group, every member of which breathes the same air, uses the same soaps — is, in short, subjected to the same environmental hazards — as all of us are. There is one outstanding exception: their nutritional preferences, member-for-member, substantially include whole grains and food made therefrom.

Many native tribesmen in Nigeria are cancer free. Their staple diet is cassava, rich in nitrilosides. Amygdalin (Laetrile) is a nitriloside. Nigerian people eat very little or no processed food. The work of Dr. Oke, of the University of Ile-Ifa, is confirmation of this observation.

The Hunzas in Pakistan commonly live to 90 and 100 years of age. Meat is a rarity consumed only several times a year. In a February 17, 1974 Parade Magazine article, "You Live to be 100 in Hunza," Senator Charles Percy comments: "Hunzukuts eat sparingly, depending on the fruits, vegetables and grains farmed in the area. Farming is organic, as it has been for 2,000 years." (There is a direct statistical correlation of increased incidence of cancer, incidentally, in the geographical location of heavy meat-eating populations.)

Dr. Ernst Krebs, Jr., makes this comment: "Western progress in agriculture has caused the abandonment of the natural vitamins. We have abandoned millet, which is rich in nitrilosides" [that body of natural substances which Krebs believes inhibit cancer cells] "and we went on to wheat. We quit eating the seeds of the common fruits as our affluence grew. The reduction in the incidence of cancer appears proportional to the amount of nitrilosides (amygdalin) included in the diet of certain geographical populations."

Many statistics can be tendered to explain the incidence or lack of cancer in a society. Chief among these are the studies linking fat and meat consumption to cancer of the bowel. Care must be taken not to misinterpret such statistics and draw erroneous conclusions. High meat and animal-fat diets are almost always deficient in whole grains and other high-fiber foods that promote a shorter intestinal tract transit time. It is when the protein products putrefy in a lazy colon that 3-methylcholanthrene, a powerful carcinogen, is formed. The possibility exists that the high lack of fiber may relate to the problem. So a lowering of meat and fat intake and an increase in fiber foods intake may be the logical answer. Recent research has also pointed to the excess-free radical formation that develops when quantities of unsaturated oil-containing foods are consumed as being, quite possibly, one of the prime factors in the genesis of cancer. The pieces of the puzzle are here; we must dilligently examine and fit them into place.

In brief, although the objective research work needed to prove the precise correlation between cancer and diet has not been completed, numerous empirical and scientific reports from historical and contemporary sources, on a worldwide basis, make a very strong hypothesis that this is the case. Logic suggests that we ignore the establishment demagogues in white coats who reject any consideration of nutrition as a cause or preventive of cancer (although many doctors as individuals resist orthodoxy) and embrace, instead, the common-sense approach of nutritional investigation.

CHAPTER 5:

Digestive System

"Wastebasket diagnosis abounds in medicine. The excuse often given by the medical profession is that a 'label' on the patients' illness saves the patients' (or their families) money in that they do not go shopping around among doctors for a cure that does not exist! However, the search for more effective treatment should never be relaxed by patient, parent or doctor."

Carl C. Pfieffer, Ph.D., M.D.

The human body derives its energy from food. The three main groups of human foods are proteins, carbohydrates and fats, assisted by vitamins and minerals. Food is broken down in the digestive process to a form which can be utilized by the body cells. This digestive system consists of the following components, illustrated in Chart 7 on page 48.

Digestion of Carbohydrates

Carbohydrate digestion is accomplished in the following stages:
1. Raw and cooked starch is converted to maltose and dextrin.
2. Maltose to glucose.
3. Sucrose (cane sugar) to glucose and fructose.
4. Lactose (milk sugar) to glucose and galactose.

Glucose, after absorption into the blood, is transported to the cell where it combines with oxygen to create energy. Excess glucose is converted to glycogen, fat or excreted from the body.

Chart 8 shows the enzymes needed in carbohydrate digestion. In stage 1, the food is mixed with ptyalin (alpha-amylase) secreted by the parotid glands. Ptyalin breaks down starches into maltose and dextrin.

Only a slight portion of the starch is broken down in the mouth. Most passes on to the stomach untouched because the food is in the mouth for such a short time; the enzyme ptyalin can not possibly work on all the starch. Partial digestion of starch in the mouth is illustrated by chewing on a piece or cracker or bread: a sweet taste indicates that the starch is being broken down into a sugar. Even though most of the starch passes into the stomach undigested, the ptyalin mixed with it continues to work for several minutes while in the stomach. Therefore, the average total digestion of starches due to ptyalin is from 30 to 40 percent; five percent occurs in the mouth and the remainder in the stomach.

Once partially-digested substances have moved on to the duodenum, they cause the pancreas to secrete pancreatic alpha-amylase to perform basically the same fuction as ptyalin in the mouth. Splitting starch into maltose and dextrin, pancreatic amylase is more powerful than ptyalin and converts almost all of the starches into maltose and dextrin.

The final stages of carbohydrate breakdown in the intestine convert sucrose into glucose and fructose. All carbohydrates are converted to one of the simple sugars: Glucose, fructose, and galactose, sorbitol, manitol, xylitol and a few other simple sugars are also present, but in very small amounts. The digestion begins in the mouth and is completed in the small intestine.

These simple sugars then pass into the blood stream. Glucose can be immediately transported to the cells for use in the energy cycle; all other sugars go through a glycogen cycle in the liver and are then converted to glucose, fat, or remain as glycogen to be stored in the muscles or liver for a time when the blood sugar drops and the body needs glucose. After fat is formed, either in the liver or in the fat cell (as triglycerides), the fuel value is less available to the body.

Chart 7
Digestive System Components

Sub-System in Digestive Process	Operation
Salivary glands	Secrete a clear alkaline fluid from glands in the mouth; the saliva moistens and softens food and contains a digestive enzyme — ptyalin — which begins the breakdown of complex starch into more simple sugars.
Stomach	An expansion of the esophagus. Secretes gastric juice, containing hydrochloric acid and digestive enzymes, primarily pepsin.
Pancreas	A gland situated behind the stomach, its secretion contains digestive enzymes and an internal hormone for regulation of carbohydrate metabolism (insulin).
Liver	A large gland which produces bile. The liver can convert simple sugars into glycogen, an inert sugar, for storage.
Gall bladder	A reservoir for bile.
Duodenum	The first section of the small intestine.
Small intestine	Portion of the alimentary canal where digestive processes are brought to completion. The area where digestive end products are absorbed into the bloodstream.
Large intestine	Last portion of the alimentary canal. Reservoir for waste products of digestion.
Rectum	Distal (furthest) portion of the alimentary canal.

Chart 8
Enzymes Needed for Carbohydrate Digestion

Enzyme	Secreted by or occurs in	Food product acted upon	Products of this enzyme reaction
Pancreatic lipase (steapsin)	Pancreas into intestine	Fats	Fatty acids, glycerol
Pepsin	Gastric juice	Protein	Proteoses and peptones
Trypsin and Chymotrypsin	(Pancreas) Intestine	Protein	Proteoses, peptones and polypeptides
Enterokinase (a peptidase)	(Pancreas) Intestine	Trypsinogen (from Pancreas)	Trypsin
Peptidases (erepsin — a group of enzymes)	(Pancreas) Intestine	Peptones, polypeptides, dipeptides	Amino acids
Nuclease — a group of enzymes	(Pancreas) Intestine	Nucleic acid & derivatives	Purine & pyrimidine bases, a sugar (carbohydrate), phosphoric acid

Glucose can combine with oxygen in the cell to form energy leaving the waste products water and carbon dioxide. It looks like this:

$$C_6 H_{12} O_6 \text{ (Glucose)} + O_2 = \text{Energy} + CO_2 \text{ and } H_2O$$

Glucose can also be converted to glycogen, an inert substance stored in the muscles and liver which can be quickly converted back to glucose. The conversions look like this:

$$\underset{\text{(Glucose)}}{C_6H_{12}O_6} - \underset{\text{(water)}}{H_2O} = \underset{\text{(glycogen)}}{C_6H_{10}O_5}$$

$$C_6H_{10}O_5 + H_2O = C_6H_{12}O_6$$

Digestion of Fats

Fats are not broken down in the human body until they reach the small intestine where there is a two-stage change:
1. Fats are emulsified by bile from the liver.
2. Emulsified fats are converted to fatty acids and glycerol, by enzymes from the pancreas.

Glycerol and fatty acids are recombined upon absorption to form neutral fat which may be oxidized to furnish energy, or may be stored as body fat for reserve energy supply or to combine with protein to form body tissue.

The enzymes required for fat digestion is lipase, secreted by the pancreas (Note: Bile must act to emulsify, i.e., breakdown to small particles, before the lipase can be really effective).

Once fat reaches the small intestine the gall bladder releases bile, a product of the liver, stored in the gall bladder. Bile has the function of emulsifying fat globules, i.e., breaking down the large fat globules taken in from our food into smaller globules. The bile does not digest the fat but only makes smaller pieces out of bigger pieces. Emulsification increases the surface area of the fat by making smaller pieces with more exposed surfaces, allowing fat-digestive enzymes of the pancreas more surface area to work on. The enzyme in this process is lipase. About 10-20 percent of the fat intake is broken down into long-chain fatty acids and glycerol, which pass into the lymphatic circulation and eventually to the liver. The remaining 80-90 percent of short chain fatty acids and glycerol go directly to the liver via the blood stream. Criteria for determining which path a fat will take depends on the size of the fat; those with shorter-chain fatty acids are absorbed directly into the blood stream.

Digestion of Protein

1. Albumin (protein) to acid metaprotein
2. Primary proteoses
3. Secondary proteoses
4. Peptones (the first dialyzable stage at which they can be absorbed)
5. Polypeptides or dipeptides
6. Peptides
7. Amino acids (the stage in which they can be assimilated).

The following enzymes are needed in protein digestion:
PEPSIN (Stomach)
PANCREATIN (Small Intestine)
1. Trypsin
2. Chymotrypsin
3. Erepsin

A protein is a long chain of many amino acids linked together by a polypeptide bond. Proteins furnish the body with amino acids, which are then made into new structural proteins according to the blueprints contained in the genes. These new structural proteins act as building blocks for almost every cellular structure of the body. Proteins in food must be broken down by a series of steps in the digestive system in the same way that carbohydrates and fats are. The small intestine cannot absorb most proteins as such, but can absorb amino acids from which they are built.

Therefore, the objective of the digestive system is to break proteins into amino acids by cleaving the peptide bonds which hold them together.

Digestion of protein does not occur before it reaches the stomach. Glands in the stomach secrete substances that are responsible for the initiation of protein digestion.

Protein is not synonomous with meat. Other excellent sources of protein are nuts, seeds, sprouts, and other non-animal sources. Americans consume an average of 193 pounds of protein per person per year, but the handling and processing of meat may be questionable. It is common practice today to reduce fattening time of cattle, chickens, pigs and lambs. Fattening is a natural biological process when animals are fed healthy diets over a period of time, but today hormones are used to reduce fattening time to quickly produce a plump animal for slaughter. Traces of these hormones may persist in the meat. There are some who recognize this problem and market hormone-free meats and certify them as such. When you buy meat for your own consumption, it would be wise to specify such brands.

Nutrition and Cancer

Two vital nutrients necessary for tumor survival as well as growth are amino acids and glucose. Amino acids are needed for protein synthesis in normal cells as well as in malignant cells. The cancer traps nitrogen from the nitrogen pool of the host for the synthesis of some of the amino acids and robs other amino acids that have already been synthesized. (This is at the expense of the normal cells.) Once the cancer cells synthesize and incorporate proteins into their structural makeup, the amino acids are not recycled as would normally occur. The direction of amino acids then becomes a one-way street, leading to the cancer cells, because of their chaotic growth rate and the negligible release of amino acids.

Glucose is the major fuel source in the body, and the basic compound into which many foods are converted. Robbing this substance from the body is certainly one of the primary ways a tumor undermines its opponent. The tumor seems to be better equipped to capture glucose than are normal cells, and acts as a glucose trap using from five to 10 times the amount that normal cells would, due to the increase in fermentation.

Most of the work on cancer cell metabolism was carried out by Otto Warburg, a two-time Nobel Prize winner. In 1931, Warburg discovered oxygen-transferring enzymes of cell respiration, and in 1944 he discovered the active groups of the hydrogen-transferring enzymes. Warburg believed that the onset of anaerobic glycolysis (air-deprived glucose formation) was the harbinger of a cancer cell. If this is true, the cause of cancer may be determined by discovering the cause for a change in metabolism, by a normal cell, to anaerobic glycolysis. In 1966, Warburg found that a 35 percent decrease in oxygen caused embryonic cells to change into cells with malignant characteristics. Based on this work, he proposed the use of vitamin E as a possible curb to the incidence of cancer. Since vitamin E reduces the cells' need for oxygen, a cell may be able to tolerate much lower levels of oxygen available to it in the presence of vitamin E without changing its metabolic patterns toward that of a cancer cell. The effectiveness of vitamin E on cancer, however, has not been proven.

The nutritional program presented in this book provides a cancer prevention program based on the requirements of the human digestive system outlined in the preceding pages, together with changes in diet and supplements of vitamins and enzymes to counteract the assault of junk foods on the system that might set the stage for cancer.

Carcinogens

There are many different carcinogens and their source varies. Some are in the water we drink, others in the food we eat and still others in the air we breathe. In present day society, the number of carcinogens entering or affecting our bodies is increasing every day. It is foolhardy to believe that, even with the most stringent environmental protection plans, we can ever decrease the carcinogen level to a safe level. Research money in large amounts is awarded each year by governmental granting agencies to identify carcinogens. Suspect carcinogens are applied to animals to determine the increase in the number of tumors. This research is valid and we should, as much as possible, eliminate contact with such known carcinogens.

However, carcinogens by themselves do not cause cancer. Even orthodox medicine finally agrees that carcinogens are only the irritant that determines the location of the lump or bump the medical establishment recognizes as cancer. In reality, these lumps and bumps are only the symptom or final manifestation of an underlying metabolic imbalance or weakness in our body's intrinsic defenses against disease. The carcinogen triggers the normal trophoblast cells within the body into rapidly-proliferating cancer cells that the body either has not protected itself from or cannot.[1]

Immune System

We do not all come down with cancer. Why not? The cancer cell does not belong in the human body. Our bodies are protected against any foreign organism or agent by an immune system. If we had an auditorium filled with people and the flu virus were to be introduced into the auditorium, not all would come down with the flu. The ones contracting the illness would be those having a low resistance to the virus.

Even when subjected to carcinogens, the immune system attempts to keep the body in a steady state. The body's normal condition is one of health. Anything that enters the system — a virus, a bacteria, or a foreign protein — causes a reaction that will lead to a rejection of the invader. The cancer cells, once formed, should be eliminated. In some instances, however — and these instances become more numerous each day as a disease progresses — the body is in so weakened a condition that the immune system fails to reject the cancer cell. When not rejected, cancer cells divide rapidly, ultimately forming the lump or bump medical science has come to recognize as cancer.

Most of us are born with an efficient immune system. But an alarming percentage of us, unfortunately, do everything we can to destroy our bodies. The foods we eat are, for the most part, highly processed; many fall into the category of junk foods or those we know to be nutritionally worthless. Excessive stress of everyday life also takes its toll — lengthy work hours with little time for recreation, play or exercise. All these factors lead to lowered efficiency in the immune system. The end result, all too often, is a metabolic or degenerative disease.

The principal mechanism of the body's defense against a foreign substance is its reserve of white blood cells, continually circulating throughout the body; they have the ability to destroy invading viruses, or even errant deviating cells if they are recognized. *The first malignant cancer cell should be destroyed right at this point!* However, science now recognizes that the cancer cell wraps itself in a protein coating having the same electrical charge as the white cells. The two identical charges, of course, repel each other. The cancer cell, in this clever protective disguise, could remain unattacked and free to proliferate, were it not for another marvelous mechanism: the enzymes (see Chapter Seven) that continuously circulate in our bloodstreams and have the ability to dissolve the protein coat from around the malignant cell. Once robbed of protective coating, the original proliferating cells are recognized and overwhelmed by white cells. This, then, is the body's intrinsic method of ridding itself of malignancies.

Thankfully, in most of us this enzymatic first line of defense will prove adequate. However, logic recognizes that different bodies will vary in their ability to function. Just as some of us have more resistance to infection than others, obviously some bodies will be more able intrinsically to protect themselves than others. What of those individuals who have perhaps inherited a weak immune system or, for reasons we will outline later, have insufficient enzymes available? Our Creator, the master engineer, has designed an extrinsic protective system in the foods available for us to eat. A perfect back-up system that could not have just happened.

It is about these foods, and their nutrients, which compose our extrinsic defense against cancer, that this book is mainly concerned.

At this point we should say you are not what you eat, but rather, what your system is able to *digest, absorb and utilize*. This explains why one person can eat junk foods and look and feel comparatively well while another can eat all the "right foods" and be sick. The well person's first line of defense (his or her remarkable body) may be better capable of deriving the nutrients needed to stay well than the well-fed sickly person. Even a well person whose orchestra of endocrine organs is capable of secreting an abundance of enzymes to utilize the nutrients in his foods will not be as well as he would have been, had he supported his body systems.

It should be stated also that while all of the nutrients necessary for sound health are available from proper diet, supplementation may, in specific cases, be required. In some situations local unavailability of foods, other illnesses, heredity, advancing age or allergy may make assimilations of total body requirements difficult to achieve. The Holistic or Metabolic physician will then recommend proper supplements; for examples, we would cite vitamin C, vitamin A, vitamin E, the trace elements, hydrochloric acid, minerals and the enzymes. Most of our necessary nutrients today have either been synthesized in the laboratory or extracted from their natural source.

A nutritionally-trained professional should be able to determine if your age or special situation requires the insurance factor of supplementation.

Notes — CHAPTER FIVE

1. For a thorough explanation of the creation and metabolism of trophoblast cells into malignancy see *"Unitarian or Trophoblastic Thesis of Cancer,"* E. T. Krebs, Jr., Ph.D..

CHAPTER 6:

The Role of Vitamins

*"The American public is being sold a bill of goods about cancer...
today the press releases coming out of the National Cancer Institute
have all the honesty of the Pentagon".*

Dr. James Watson, Nobel Prize winner

Vitamins are organic substances contained in foods in minute
quantities. They are both fundamental and essential for the
well-being and healthy operation of our bodies.

Identification and isolation of vitamins is comparatively recent,
beginning only in this century. Our knowledge is still far from
complete, although we do know that human need for certain
nutrients has increased tremendously because of such factors as
pollution, stress, increased consumption of refined foods, etc.
While most animals can create their own vitamin C, man cannot.
It is more likely that each of our diets is deficient in one or
more vitamins and just as likely that we are unaware of this
vitamin deficiency. Protection is simple — adjust our diet as close
to that of nature as possible, include in our diet unrefined and
unprocessed natural foods, and supplement those nutrients in
which we may be deficient.

Table of Vitamins

Vitamins are designated by letters and subscripts. Chart 9 lists
known vitamins with a letter designation, name of the specific
compound and its function in the human body. Those vitamins of

most vital importance in the prevention and treatment of cancer are described in the text.

Chart 9
TABLE OF VITAMINS

VITAMIN Chemical Properties (stability)	BIOLOGICAL FUNCTION
VITAMIN A — Carotene fat soluble; stable to heat; unstable to air; destroyed by ultraviolet	Essential for growth of young; increases resistance to urinary and respiratory infection; lactation and reproduction; night vision (visual purple); proper appetite and digestion; skin health.
VITAMIN D — Calciferol fat soluble; stable to light, heat and air	Absorption and metabolism of calcium and phosphorus; clotting; heat action; and proper gland and nerve function; tooth and bone formation; skin respiration
VITAMIN E — Tocopherol stable to visible light, heat, acid & alkali; destroyed by u.v. light; rancid fats reduce its potency	Blood flow to heart; fertility; lung protection; male potency; prevents toxemia of pregnancy; pituitary regulation; reduces blood cholesterol; retards aging
VITAMIN K — Menadione Fat soluble	Blood clotting (prevents hemorrhage); vital for normal liver function; vitality and longevity factor
VITAMIN B_1 — Thiamine Water soluble; unstable to ultraviolet; destroyed by boiling in acidic solution, heat	Absorption and digestion; appetite; blood building; carbohydrate metabolism; corrects and prevents beriberi; learning ability; promotes growth, resistance to infection and proper nerve function
VITAMIN B_2 — Riboflavin water soluble; stable to air, heat; unstable to visible light, u.v.; destroyed by alkalies	Antibody and red blood cell formation; aids iron assimilation and protein metabolism; healthy skin and digestive tract; prolongs life; promotes growth and general health; vision
VITAMIN B_3 — Niacin water soluble; stable to heat; light, air, acid and alkali	Circulation; hormone (sex) production; growth; hydrochloric acid production; maintenance of nervous system; metabolism; reduces cholesterol level; respiration
VITAMIN B_5 — Pantothenic Acid water soluble; unstable to heat; destroyed by acid & alkali (vinegar — baking soda)	Antibody formation; carbohydrate metabolism; growth stimulation; healthy skin and nerves; maintains blood sugar level; stimulates adrenals; vitamin utilization
VITAMIN B_6 — Pyridoxine water soluble; stable in heat; unstable in light	Antibody formation; controls level of magnesium in blood and tissues; digestion; maintains sodium/potassium balance; cholesterol levels; metabolism of fats
VITAMIN B_{12} — Cyarocobalamin water soluble	Appetite; blood cell formation; cell longevity; normal metabolism of nerve tissue; protein; fat and carbohydrate metabolism, glandular and nervous system
VITAMIN B_{15} — Pangamic Acid water soluble	Cell oxidation and respiration; stimulates glucose, fat, protein metabolism, glandular and nervous system

BIOTIN, Vitamin H water soluble; stable to heat; inactivated by oxidation; synthesized by intestinal bacteria	Growth; lipid synthesis in liver; metabolism of carbohydrates; fats; protein, vit. B utilization
CHOLINE water soluble	Health of liver, kidney and nervous tissue; prevents gall stones; with inositol is basic consti- tuent of lecithin; utilization of fats
FOLIC ACID water soluble; destroyed by heat and light	Aids liver performance; appetite; cell reproduc- tion; growth; HCL production; protein metabo- lism; red blood cell formation
INOSITOL water soluble	Brain cell nutrition; fat metabolism; growth and survival of cells in bone marrow, eye and intes- tines; hair health; lecithin formation; reduces blood cholesterol; protects liver, kidney and heart
PABA — Para Aminobenzoic Acid water soluble	Blood cell formation; hair pigment; stimulates intestinal bacteria to form folic acid; protein metabolism; sun-screen
VITAMIN C — Ascorbic Acid water soluble; stable to heat; destroyed by oxygen, u.v., copper & iron cooking vessels, pasteuri- zation; canning; insecticide	Appetite, blood vessel health; calcium diffusion; prevents vitamin oxidation; promotes growth and healing; proper bone and tooth formation; pro- tects heart; raises resistance to infection; red blood cell formation
VITAMIN P — Bioflavonoids water soluble; occurs with vitamin C showing similar chemical properties	Alters permeability of capillaries; increases resis- tance to colds and flu; maintains healthy connec- tive tissue and blood vessel walls; proper absorp- tion of Vit. C; strengthens capillary walls

Vitamin A

Discovered in 1909 and synthesized in 1946, vitamin A is a fat-soluble alcohol known as retinol, and is found in natural form only in animals. Fish liver, for example, is a prime source of vitamin A with up to 300 mg of retinol per hundred grams of liver. Calf liver contains about 15-150 mg per 100 grams. Eggs, milk and butter contain only minute amounts of vitamin A. The U.S. government daily requirement allowance is set at 5,000 IU (International Units) per day for a moderately active male. Although the government states that anything over 10,000 is highly toxic, experience and statistics do not bear this out. There are, for example, 11,000 IU of vitamin A in a carrot and 43,000 IU in an average size piece of liver.

Lack of vitamin A has a known effect on animals: in general, loss of appetite, inhibited growth and an increased susceptibility to infection. Substantial deficiencies of A can lead to death. Dry and scaly skin are surface effects of a deficiency. Deficiency can also result in infection of the respiratory or urinary tract.

Most previous clinical testing of vitamin A in cancer treatment has been done in Germany, where emulsified vitamin A was used either alone or with emulsified vitamin E in conjunction with irradiation treatment. In a paper presented at the Mexican Cancer Congress on September 30, 1971 in Mexico City, Hoefer-Janker, et al, reported an effect on malignant tumors with large doses of emulsified vitamin A. This megavitamin treatment with emulsified A enhances the anti-tumor effect of radiation, alkylating agents, and enzyme therapy. Clinics in Germany are now using the megadose vitamin A therapy with positive results, especially in squamous cell carcinoma. Vitamin A alone has effected a complete remission of squamous cell carcinoma of the skin. In the same paper, Hoefer-Janker, et al, stated that much less radiation is needed with megadoses of emulsified vitamin A.

The amounts of emulsified vitamin A used in the German clinics were 300,000 IU of A daily, increased by 150,000 IU per day up to 3 million per day and continued until 60 million units had been administered. Minor adverse effects are a flakiness of the skin, especially at the mucous membranes, and sometimes headaches. More than 35,000 German patients have received this treatment without any severe side effects attributable to the emulsified vitamin A.

Dr. Hoefer-Janker presented his work on vitamin A in tumor therapy at Salzburg on April 12, 1972, sponsored by the Institute of Cancer Research, Vienna University. By then he had treated 1149 cancer patients at the Janker Clinic with megadoses of vitamin A. Standard irradiation and chemotherapy were also used. No patients died due to vitamin A intoxication even though the doses ranged from 15 to 180 million IU of vitamin A.

Vitamin A absorption occurs in the small intestine. In animals, vitamin A is ingested usually in the form of its ester, called retinal palmitate. Not all vitamin A in the oil reaches the liver, the storage organ for vitamin A. (About 90 percent of vitamin A is stored in the liver.)

To avoid the problem of a toxic liver resulting from high amounts of vitamin A (a high amount would be between 300,000 and 3 million IU per day), vitamin A for cancer treatment is used in a water-soluble (emulsified) substance. This allows for rapid and complete absorption into the lymph system and then into the blood.

More recently, Harold Manner, Ph.D., has conducted a series of tests with vitamin A on mice with tumors. In the initial tests, each experimental mouse received amygdalin injected intramuscularly in the rump area, plus 333,333 IU per kilogram of body weight of emulsified vitamin A. An enzyme preparation was designed for intratumoral use, and contained enzymes from the pea, lentil, papaya, calf thymus and beef pancreas. These enzymes were injected into and around the tumor mass every other day.

"The results were dramatic," Dr. Manner reports. "At the beginning of the experiment, tumors measured 4 to 6 mm in diameter. On the fourth day, a small white pimple developed at the site of the tumor, and in two more days the pimple ruptured and a white pus emerged. This pus was placed on a microscope slide and sent to pathologists for examination, and identified as dead tumor cells. As the pus continued to drain, tumors became smaller. In four to six weeks the tumors were completely gone on 90 percent of the 84 experimental animals. Tumors on the other 10 percent of the mice were in regression at the close of the experiment. Animals with completely regressed tumors were autopsied by the pathologist. No sign of the tumor remained."

Dr. Manner wishes us to emphasize that the enzyme and vitamin A injections have not, as yet, been clinically adopted. The results, however, are interesting and indicative of further research.

The anti-tumor characteristics of vitamin A were further investigated in a later series of tests at Loyola University to study and evaluate the leucogenic effect on non-tumorous C3H/HeJ mice. There was a significant increase in total white blood count and the differential lymphocyte counts after administration of vitamin A. At a dosage of 333,333 IU/kgm of body weight,

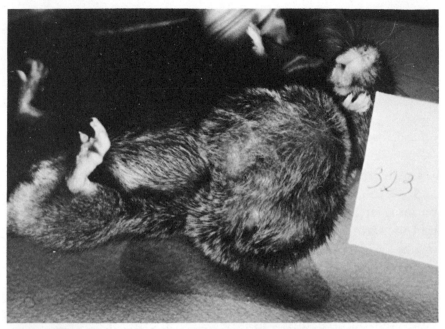

One of Dr. Manner's test animals with large tumor.

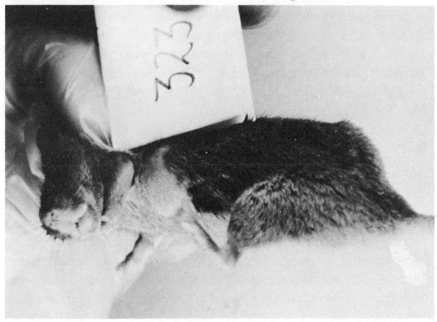

Six weeks later after amygdalin, vitamin A and enzyme treatment.

vitamin A administered orally increased the number of white blood cells from 5744.85 + 281.04 to 7374.50 + 289.48.

The focus of research is now on combined use of vitamin A, amygdalin and enzymes (discussed in a later chapter).

Vitamin C

Probably the most important factor in determining the progress and outcome of any cancer case is the natural resistance of the patient. Orthodox cancer treatments would be vastly improved if methods were used to enhance natural resistance. Increasing the intake of vitamin C (ascorbic acid, sodium ascorbate, calcium ascorbate) has this effect. In many cancer patients, ascorbate improves the state of well-being, as measured by improved appetite, increased mental alertness, decreased requirement for pain-controlling drugs, and other clinical criteria.

The most important work has been carried out by Ewan Cameron, M.D., chief surgeon in Vale of Leven Hospital, Loch Lomonside, Scotland. An account of his work, entitled "Supplemental Ascorbate in the Supportive Treatment of Cancer: Prolongation of Survival Times in Terminal Human Cancer," was published in the October, 1976, issue of *Proceedings of the National Academy of Sciences U.S.A.*

Clinical trials were begun by Cameron in Vale of Leven Hospital in November 1971, and several reports on these trials have been published. In the main study, 100 patients with advanced cancer received vitamin C (sodium ascorbate), in amounts of 10 grams per day, and compared with 100 control patients who were matched for sex, age, and type of cancer and were treated in the same way, except for ascorbate, in the same hospital. The average survival time of the ascorbate-treated patients was over four times that of the controls, and a fraction of these patients have had very long survival times, over 20 times the average for the controls, and no longer show signs of malignant disease.

The U.S. medical cancer establishment has turned a blind eye to these promising vitamin C results.

Some highly significant vitamin C work has been undertaken in recent years under the direction of Arthur B. Robinson, Ph.D. at the Linus Pauling Institute in Menlo Park, California. Dr. Robinson states that the data shows vitamin C, in very high doses, is startlingly effective in reducing the incidence and severity of skin cancer in laboratory mice.

Cancer was induced by daily ultraviolet radiation of hairless mice that lived throughout the experiments on the designated diets. At dosages comparable to 100 grams of vitamin C per day, it was decreased about five-fold. A diet restricted to apples, pears, carrots, tomatoes, wheat grass, sunflower seeds and bananas decreased the cancer by about the same amount as the very high vitamin C dosages. When used together, the raw fruits and vegetables and vitamin C caused a remarkable 35-fold decrease in cancer incidence.

"The incidence of severe lesions in these experiments," Dr. Robinson's findings explain, "was caused to vary over a 70-fold range by nutritional measures alone. Regardless of the specific nutrition or the specific cancer assay system used, this result supports the view that optimum nutrition should be given a high priority in cancer research."

Dr. Bob Cathcart, in treating over 12,000 patients with massive doses of vitamin C, has developed a guideline for practical application which he refers to as the "bowel tolerance" concept. The California physician has successfully treated viral pneumonia, mononucleosis, "flu", colds, hepatitis, shingles, and cold sores with this method. He has never had to intern a patient with a viral disease in the hospital, occasionally administering vitamin C intravenously in his office.

Dr. Cathcart found that the individual's own body will determine how much vitamin C it requires. The cut-off point is determined by the occurrence of diarrhea. In an interview in the May, 1979 issue of *Public Scrutiny*, Cathcart stated, "The tolerance level in each individual differs. Some days you can tolerate more — some days less — but from general experience I label a cold as a 20- to 30-gram cold, or 60-gram flu, according to how much a person can take before he reaches the bowel tolerance level."

Cathcart stressed that inadequate doses of C may be useless in treating virus-related diseases. If a cold is treated with two or even 20 grams of C, the cold may linger. "With bad colds or influenza we do not seem to shorten the duration of the infection but we render patients asymptomatic (relatively free from symptoms) so they can weather the disease without the headaches, stuffy nose or generally lousy feeling the accompanies such problems." The vitamin C will permeate every cell of the body before it reaches the bowel, according to Dr. Cathcart. He justified these massive doses by explaining further that the sick cell is using vitamin C at a tremendous rate because there are toxins put out by the viruses within the sick cell rendering it scorbutic (with scurvy).

In short, if you have not reached bowel tolerance (diarrhea), you have not taken enough vitamin C.

These intriguing results obviously demand further research but the federal government has been consistently unwilling to finance major work into the relationship between nutrition and disease. This prompted Arthur Robinson and associates to run a unique series of advertisements in the *Wall Street Journal*.

While at the Pauling Institute Dr. Art Robinson, the co-founder of the Institute, applied for NCI grants of a paltry $50,000 based on the work of Dr. Ewan Cameron. The prestigious institute was refused funds for their work on five different occasions.

Vitamin B15 (Pangamic Acid)

Pangamic acid, a vitamin discovered by Dr. E. T. Krebs, Jr., has been under scientific investigation resulting in widespread use in the U.S.S.R. for many years. It is probably the vitamin supplement most often required since its chief sources, such as rice bran, are not included in American diets.

Trained nutritionists, among whom can be numbered too few medically trained doctors, recognize the tremendous asset this vitamin is to cell metabolism. The contribution of B15 or pangamic acid to physical fitness and body endurance is inestimable. In the specific instance of cancer, the increased blood oxygenation provided by vitamin B15 precludes the low oxygen environment which enables malignancy to flourish.

Vitamin E

The exact role of vitamin E in body metabolism has not been determined. However, it is apparent that since vitamin E reduces need for oxygen, a cell may be able to endure low levels of oxygen changing its metabolic pattern toward malignancy.

Vitamin B17 (Amygdalin)

Developed by Drs. E. T. Krebs, Sr. and Jr., amygdalin is the crown jewel in the extrinsic nutritional defense mechanism against cancer. Just as it is not the purpose of this book to expound at length on the Unitarian Trophoblastic Thesis of Cancer, neither is it our intention to dwell on the metabolic pathway of amygdalin other than in a rudimentary explanation.

The word "amygdalin" comes from the Greek "amygdale," or almond. Amygdalin was first found in bitter almonds, and its taste resembles almonds. Amygdalin was first used by a Chinese herbalist (Pen T' Sao) in the year 2800 B.C. and has been in use since that time, making nonsense of the FDA claim it is a "new drug" and requires FDA approval.

Amygdalin is a cyanogenetic glycoside that occurs naturally in over 1100 edible plants, grasses and seeds. Our most easily accessible sources are the seeds of the Rosaceae plant family —apricots, peaches, plums, prunes, bitter almonds, cherries, apples — and a number of lentils and grasses. Other amygdalin-containing foods are millet, cassava, maize, sorghum, field bean, lima bean, bamboo, sugar cane, kidney bean, sweet potato, lettuce, linseed and almond. Amygdalin is one of a family of cyanide-containing substances collectively referred to as nitrilosides. These cyanide-producing, sugar-containing compounds are naturally occurring compounds and have a physiological or protective function. The cassava plant contains these compounds throughout its system, with the richest concentration in the root.

Ingested amygdalin is enzymatically broken down in the intestinal tract by way of bacterially-produced beta-glucosidase. The resultant prunasin, mandelonitrile, and other constituents travel via the blood to the liver where they are converted to the corresponding glucuronide.

The basic concept of the glucuronides as a protective mechanism against the systemically-toxic side effects of orthodox chemotherapy has been known for many years. Recent clinical observations by Drs. Mario Soto, Paul Wedel and Donald Cole continue to indicate that when they administer mixed therapy using chemotherapeutic drugs combined with amygdalin the side effects of these drugs are vastly reduced.

For over 40 years, science has recognized that cancers contain a level of an enzyme called beta-glucuronidase many times higher than those of normal cells. The beta-glucuronidase of the cancer cell has the unique enzymatic ability to cleave active, deadly cyanide from the cyanogenic glucuronide molecule released by the liver into the blood, thus triggering its own destruction. Normal cells without the cleaving enzyme remain unharmed.

We wish to emphasize that the cyanide as contained in natural occurring amygdalin is benign and totally nontoxic until it reaches the malignancy, where the cancer cell's singular ability to unlock the poison, cyanide, assists the white cells in its own destruction.

With the exception of the suppressed Sloan-Kettering experiments, modern research is notable for its lack of interest in the nutritional approach to cancer control. Yet, established medicine is well aware of scientific criteria and quotes them at length in attacking the use of amygdalin.*

*For example, California State Board of Public Health - **Quackery And The Cancer Law.**

We repeat the scientific axiom fundamental to all scientific research, i.e., that a negative proposition cannot be proven. In other words, it is unscientific for orthodox medical practitioners to make the statement that no diet containing amygdalin prevents cancer. This is a negative statement impossible of scientific proof and is the total antithesis of the empirical evidence of effective clinical usage by metabolic physicians, which is ignored by biased establishment researchers.

What is Laetrile? — Origin and Development

The isolation of amygdalin is a simple extractive procedure. First the kernels or seeds are defatted with ether. Then this fat-free residue is boiled in alcohol, filtered and cooled. The amygdalin is the white crystaline substance that is separated from other compounds existing naturally in seeds during the cooling and filtering process.

Robiquet and Boutron, in France, first isolated crystalline amygdalin in 1830. Although many cyanogenic glycosides exist, they are, at most, amygdalin-like. There is one, and only one, true amygdalin with a chemical specification.[1]

In 1952, Ernst Krebs, Jr., altered the amygdalin molecule synthetically "to make the empirical apricot formula safe for administration to humans." This new compound was patented and called Laetrile®. Unlike amygdalin, it contains glucuronic acid in place of glucose. Therefore, Laetrile®, with a capital 'L' and a registered patent mark, was not originally a synonym for amygdalin since it was not plain amygdalin, which does not contain a molecule of glucose. Laetrile is a synthetic derivative of glucuronic acid and, therefore, is designated as a glucuronide. Laetrile was developed at the John Beard Memorial Foundation of San Francisco. It was patented in 1958 by Ernst Krebs, Sr. and Ernst Krebs, Jr. (Brit Pat. 788,855). It is laevorotary (turns polarized light to the left as does amygdalin). Krebs combined the first three letters of the word laevorotary, and the last five letters of the word, nitrile, and coined the trade name Laetrile®. As Laetrile® became more popular, the word was borrowed by some when referring to any glycosidic compound containing cyanide and exhibiting this laevorotary power.

In reality, most research and clinical work today uses amygdalin. The glucuronide Laetrile® is very scarce and presently its cost is prohibitive. Narrowing the use of such compounds down to basically one substance does minimize the confustion experienced in previous years. However, the importance of knowing the exact structure and purity of any compound tested cannot be stressed enough. Lack of this knowledge in the past has lead to an array of results which are extremely contradictory and ultimately useless.

A prime reason for inconsistent results in therapy has been that, until recently — and since the time of the original amygdalin production at the Krebs and Delmar Laboratories — there has been a lack of consistently high extracting and packaging standards among the various amygdalin manufacturers. It is certainly not that the technical definition and specifications for Laetrile® amygdalin has not been exacting enough. For over 150 years, these standards were defined in all scientific literature, including the authoritatively-definitive Merck Index. Part of the problem was the extreme instability of amygdalin, once extracted and placed in an aqueous solution. Once in water, unless heavily and unnaturally buffered, amygdalin degrades into subpotency and therapeutically inactive forms. Suffice it to say here amygdalin should never, despite various suppliers' claims of stabilization, be purchased or used from a liquid solution of unknown age. Only pure natural crystalline amygdalin is acceptable. For a more scholarly discourse, read *The Extraction And Packaging of Therapeutically Effective Amygdalin,* included in the Appendix of this book.

Notes — CHAPTER SIX

1. See "The Extraction Identification and Packaging of Thera-peutically Effective Amygdalin", Appendix VII.

CHAPTER 7:

The Role of Enzymes In Cancer Treatment

"If you will tell the utter, absolute truth, it is remarkable how most of your problems are solved. It simplifies life tremendously. If you start telling half the truth or three-quarters of the truth, they will get you."

Dr. Dean Burk, former head,
Cytochemistry Department, National
Cancer Institute, and one of its
original founders

Enzymes are catalysts — specifically proteins, of which there are more than two thousand varieties altogether — that play a vital role in every human physical function. Three enzymes are instrumental in the use of amygdalin (vitamin B17) in cancer therapy: beta-glucosidase, beta-glucuronidase, and rhodanase.

Historically, enzyme therapy has been used in cancer therapy many times. Some physicians have been able to obtain beneficial results, while others, due to the enzymes' non-selective proteolytic property, have not. Since the early enzyme-therapy experimentation (1900-1915), various enzyme complexes have been synthesized, many of which exhibit a certain specificity for cancerous tissue.

The most important role of the enzyme complex may be digestion of the protein coat, leaving the tumor open to attack by the body's natural white cell defenses. If this is true, chemotherapeutic drugs, irradiation, cyanide from amygdalin, and the action of vitamin A all have a greater anti-tumor effect when used in conjunction with the enzyme complex.

The pancreas produces digestive enzymes that break down food. These enzymes are secreted in the form of precursors and active enzymes. The precursors are trypsinogen and chymotrypsinogen which convert to their active forms of trypsin and chymotrypsin in the presence of enterokinase, found in the duodenum, and in the presence of trypsin, respectively. These are proteolytic enzymes that break down proteins to polypeptides and amino acids. Two enzymes — pancreatic amylase, which breaks down polysaccharides to disaccharides, and lipase, which converts neutral triglycerides to diglycerides, monoglycerides and free fatty acids — are secreted in their active forms; in this respect, they are unlike trypsin and chymotrypsin, which are secreted in their inactive forms.

Well over 70 years ago, London and New York doctors noted that injections of trypsin had an anti-cancer effect. This was reported extensively in the medical journals of the time. It is worth recording here a selection of these medical reports because their existence casts a dark shadow of doubt over the motivation of our modern medical establishment. The considerable anti-tumor effect of enzymes, reported so long ago, is today ignored. In fact, enzyme proponents are scorned and persecuted. Why?

Following is a selective listing of these early medical research reports on the anti-tumor effects of enzymes and related treatments and research. The italicized comments on some of the articles are by embryologist John Beard and were published in 1911.

1. Rice, Clarence C.: "Treatment of Cancer of the Larynx by Subcutaneous Injections of Pancreatic Extract (Trypsin)." *Medical Record,* New York, November 24, 1906, pp. 812-816.

2. Wiggin, Frederick H.: "Case of Multiple Fibro-Sarcoma of the Tongue." *Journal of the American Medical Association,* December 15, 1906, pp. 2003-2006. *Nine months later the patient was examined by two hospital physicians, found free*

from malignant disease, and considered cured. A copy of their certificate is in the writer's [Beard's] possession.

3. Golley, F. B.: "Two Cases of Cancer Treated by the Injection of Pancreatic Extract." *Medical Record,* New York, December 8, 1906, pp. 918-919.

4. Golley, F. B.: "Two Cases of Cancer Treated with Trypsin." Supplementary report to the foregoing in *Medical Record,* May 8, 1909, pp. 804-805.

At the above date the one patient was in "fairly good health", the other — apparently a "scirrhus" cancer of the bowel —died in "the summer of 1908"... "Treatment by injection of trypsin was continued at intervals up to June, 1907." There was "not much pain up to the last three months. The suffering was nothing like that usually experienced in such cases."

Other very favorable points are noted in the report — such as that an artificial anus never became necessary, and *"the character of the disease changed from an active and rapidly progressive type to a slow and practically stationary one, which not only prolonged life, but shut off the disease from outside irritative influences, making life more bearable and wholesome by the formation of membrane over the raw surfaces: in short, replacing an active loathsome disease by one more durable."*

In the light of our knowledge of today, the treatment in this case was carried out with preparations much too weak for their task, and probably far too little amylopsin was employed.

5. Campbell, James T.: "Trypsin Treatment of Malignant Disease (Left Tonsil, Base of Tongue, Epiglottis)." *Journal of the American Medical Association,* January 19, 1907, pp. 225-226.

6. Geoth, Richard A.: "Pancreatic Treatment of Cancer with Report of a Cure." *Journal of the American Medical Association,* March 23, 1907, p. 1030.

7. Duprey, H.: "Trypsin in Epithelioma of Larynx." *New Orleans Medical and Surgical Journal,* vol. 68, p. 33.

8. Cutfield, A.: "Trypsin Treatment in Malignant Disease." *British Medical Journal,* August 31, 1907, p. 525.

9. Donati: "The Trypsin Treatment of Malignant Disease." (Review of Medicine), *British Medical Journal,* March 2, 1907. (Recurrent sarcoma of testicle.)

10. Marsden, Aspinall: "Carcinoma of Cervix Uteri successfully treated with the Pancreatic Ferment." *General Practitioner,* January 11, 1908, p. 22.

11. Meggit, Henry: "The Pancreatic Treatment of Cancer." *General Practitioner,* March 21, 1908. (Cure in seven months of recurrent cancer in liver.)

12. Franklin, Byjay, Tirelee, Ritnin: "Correct Approach to Cancer Therapy." *Lotta Workana Research,* March 8, 1908, p. 381. (Reduction of pain in rectal and visceral areas with oral enzyme and ancillary therapies substituted for conventional treatment.)

Note the dates — 1906, 1907, 1908, 1909 — all over seventy years ago!! Today enzymatic treatment of cancer is totally rejected by our medical establishment. The American Cancer Society, the American Medical Association and the FDA dismiss such treatments as "quackery". Why? Obviously not because enzymes are unsuccessful. The fear of extensive testing of enzyme treatments suggests that segments of our medical establishment are only too aware that cancer can be prevented. Failure to recognize a simple, cheap preventive exposes certain segments of the orthodox medical establishment as callous charlatans, trading profit for people's lives. So we need to ask the question: who *are* the quacks? Who *are* the charlatans?

The Manner Research at Loyola University

In recent years, this early research on enzymes has been picked up, expanded and verified by researchers abroad or outside the AMA-ACS-FDA establishment. In the 1960s and '70s several investigators confirmed the anti-tumor effects of vitamin A. In 1971, Dr. Hoefer-Janker in Germany demonstrated that 40 percent of tumors injected with enzyme preparations showed a positive regression. In 1973, Tiscjer, et al, treated 119 patients with enzyme preparations and found that cancer disappeared in 47 percent of the cases.

In 1978, supported by funds from outside the medical establishment, Dr. Harold Manner, Chairman of the Department of Biology at Loyola University in Chicago, undertook anti-tumor experiments using a combined therapy: amygdalin, vitamin A and enzyme complex. In this test 550 C3H/HeJ breeder mice were divided into 11 groups of 50 animals each. C3H/HeJ retired breeder female mice were used because about 80 percent spontaneously develop malignant mammary tumors between 12 and 17 months of age.

The application of this combined treatment resulted in an 89.3 percent complete remission rate and 100 percent regression rate of various degrees. The rationale was: the enzyme complex attacks the tumor directly and digests the surrounding protein coat, allowing the amygdalin, vitamin A, and the body's immune system to fight the cancer. Dr. Manner followed this with an experiment to determine the effects of each substance individually; the findings confirm that a combined metabolic treatment is the effective treatment, not administration of any one substance by itself. Manner summarized his findings in 1978 as follows:

"The animal tests that we conducted with funds from the Memorial Library fund of the National Health Federation are just about complete.

"The indications are that the enzymes alone do little more than retard the rate of growth of the primary tumor mass. Vitamin A by itself, and the laetrile, by itself, do not do anything that we can discern. In other words, the tumor does not slow down in its rate of growth.

"Now when the enzymes and vitamin A are used together we get a more severe retardation of tumor growth, but again, never a regression. When we add laetrile to it, we get a retardation that ends with the total regression of the tumor."

How Do Enzymes Attack Cancer?

Several theories have been proposed to explain the action of the enzyme complex, with its selective destruction of cancer. It may well be that a normal functioning pancreas, adequately producing protealytic enzymes, is the body's best defense against cancer.

This observation has been verified by Drs. Tilscher and Wrba of the Cancer Research Institute of the University of Vienna in Austria, as well as by Dr. Hoefer-Janker in Germany.

G. Stojanows, who tested the toxicity of enzymes, stated that "all tests led to the conclusion that the mixture of (protolase) can be regarded as completely atoxis" (without toxicity). He also observed there was no damage to healthy tissues and that animal experiments essentially agree with observations made at the clinic on cancer patients.

"The best way to attack cancer is to act before it starts, through the use of raw foods and vitamin supplements. The use of enzymes from these foods or food supplements should not be limited to the treatment of degenerative disease, but also used as protection for those who wish to forestall degenerative diseases."

A combination of beef pancreas, calf thymus, and extract of the garden pea, the lentil bean, and the papaya has been found by Dr. Manner to be the most destructive force against the cancer and/or the protein coat surrounding the cancer cell. Once the protein coat is dissolved, cancer cells can actually be said to be defenseless. The enzymes in the complex are fractionated hyrolysates of the beef pancreas, calf thymus, pisum sativum, lens esculenta and papyotin.

The mode of action of the components most widely used in enzyme therapy are:

Chymotrypsin - reduces inflammation.

Trypsin - digests necrotic tissue.

Amylase - digests starch.

Lipase - digests fat.

Papain - de-shields tumor tissue.

Bromelain - digest protein.

Pancreatin - natural synergistic enzyme mixture.

Thymus substance - contains enzymes.

Emulsified vitamin A - activates lysosomes and nourishes epithelium.

Emulsified vitamin E - antioxidant and cell protectant.

In addition to being a primary defense mechanism against malignant cells in the bloodstream, the pancreatic enzymes break down and aid in the digestion of the protein in our food. If heredity has provided a normal pancreas there will ordinarily be enough enzymes produced to fulfill both functions. However, a diet that requires the use of all the pancreatic enzymes for digestion may not have sufficient freely-circulating enzymes to prevent cancer. Unfortunately, a large percentage of people are genetically not able to produce enough enzymes for proper digestion, leaving no leftover enzyme for adequate defense against cancer.

Part of the metabolic approach to cancer therapy is to reduce consumption of beef or even avoid eating it entirely. The protein of beef is difficult for the pancreatic enzymes to break down and, therefore, requires a large quantity of enzymes, whereas the protein of chicken and fish is far more easily digested. The less demand we make on pancreatic enzymes to digest our food intake, the more enzymes there will be to function as part of our immune defense.

Note — CHAPTER SEVEN

1. John Beard, *The Enzymes Treatment of Cancer,* (Chatoo & Windus, London 1911), pp. 274-5.

CHAPTER 8:

Alternatives to Surgery

"Internal Medicine was born of witchcraft... surgery is a child of the battlefield."

Dr. Norman Schumway

What can one do? Statistics indicate that cancer will strike one of every four Americans during their lifetimes.

Obviously, a thorough investigation of the medical establishment is long overdue. Unless an aroused electorate puts sufficient pressure on the Congress we may well wait a couple more decades before a sluggish government raises enough courage to probe the American Cancer Society, the American Medical Association, the National Cancer Institute, Memorial Sloan-Kettering Institute, and their bureaucratic allies in the Food and Drug Administration. Meantime, the potential cancer victim must take the solution into his own hands.

Legislatures in two states, namely Massachusetts and California, have actually felt it necessary to pass laws making it mandatory that a medical doctor fully inform a patient with breast cancer of all of the alternative protocols of treatment.

Unfortunately, laws cannot be passed that would force the physician to become knowledgeable about all the alternatives. Most doctors are not only unfamiliar with the new and contradictory techniques of surgery and radiation within their own field but are hopelessly uninformed, as well, in the preventive/corrective disciplines of immunotherapy and clinical nutrition.

77

Experimental Systemic Poisons

In a previous chapter, we discussed the toxic dangers of chemotherapeutic drugs that are, at best, experimental non-specific poisons, the ill-effects of which often surpass the ravages of the disease and invariably suppress the immune system. The expected results from such lethal poisons has been compared to medical witchcraft. For further comparisons of current consensus medicine attitudes against the protocol and treatment advocated by holistic, metabolically-informed physicians, we should briefly discuss the art (as opposed to science) of surgery in its attack on cancer. In so doing, we concede that where the body's natural immune system has been neglected to the point of allowing tumor growth to affect the vital functions of an internal organ, the trauma to the body of surgery cannot be avoided. Mechanical removal of the obstruction then is imperative. But what of the patient whose vital functions are not affected?

An attempt to review the controversies and contradictions throughout the field of oncological surgery would be impossible. For the sake of brevity we will restrict ourselves to breast cancer, the most common malignancy in women and the one we are most often asked to comment upon.

Orthodoxy has traditionally regarded radical surgery as the treatment of choice; this, despite the devastating physical and psychological side effects and the indications, from the inception of the procedure, that the irreversible results do not warrant the trauma.

Until the late 1800s, breast cancer was far less incidental than at the present time. No consistent form of therapy was practiced or recognized. Patients seldom saw their doctors until the malignancy was well advanced.

During the late 1880s, William Halstead, M.D., of the Johns Hopkins University Hospital devised the radical mastectomy. In 1902, Dr. Halstead published the results of 133 operations. Although the survival rate was little better than of untreated patients, the surgical bandwagon was rolling, using as its excuse the fact that the tumors seldom recurred in the surgically treated area. The fact that the area had become surgical offal (waste parts) seems to have escaped consideration — as well as the even then recognized fact that tumor recurrences on the chest were not the usual cause of death which results primarily from metastases (spreading to the lungs, liver and other internal organs).

Halstead's operation was based on the theory that cancer was a local disease — one that spread in a predictable way, first to the lymph vessels and nodes, which for a time would act as a defense barrier until they were overwhelmed, then on to adjoining organs and tissues. This theory held, first of all, that cancer was an independent entity against which the body had no defense mechanism and, secondly, that it did not spread specifically by way of the blood.

Based upon this theory the best way to prevent spread of the disease was to excise it while it was still localized. The more extensive the operation, including lymph system, pectoral muscles, etc., the greater the chance of intercepting all tumor cells. But what if the patient still died when the disease manifested itself in a vital internal organ? The convenient explanation was that either the operation had not been extensive enough or had been performed too late. We refer to this as the "too bad — I guess we did not get it all" theory of cancer therapy.

Believe it or not, this illogical and already discredited procedure was the basis upon which generations of physicians continued to repeat surgical mayhem, notwithstanding the fact it was statistically proven to have had small value from the very beginning.

Until the mid 1950s, the possibility that the blood could serve as the route for metastases received little, if any, consideration. Unquestionably, the surgery performed during these years did as much to spread or metastasize the malignancy by way of the blood as to localize it. As short a time as 10 years ago, all physicians would have recommended, in diagnosing breast malignancy, that the entire breast be sacrificed, regardless of the stage or condition of the disease.

Only a few physicians, notably George Crile, Jr., M.D., of Cleveland Clinic and Vera Peters, M.D., of Princess Margaret

Hospital in Toronto, Canada, would have dissented, based on their practical experience that many patients could be offered far less drastic surgery without affecting survival statistics. Traditional surgical opinion refused to be swayed by their clinincal observations.

In 1955, Drs. Edwin R. Fisher and Rupert Trunbull discovered cancer cells in the blood. This was confirmed shortly thereafter by other investigators, spurring Dr. Fisher to continue investigation of tumor metastases. Unfortunately, the surgical grip on the female breast remained so firm that radical mastectomies continued, despite contradictory research questioning their value.

The continuing work of Dr. Fisher and his brother, Dr. Bernard Fisher, has ultimately resulted in orthodoxy's recognition of a fact logic should have made obvious decades before: the blood stream, not just the lymph system, is an important route for the cancer cell. We hasten to inject that the researchers still failed to recognize or investigate the possibility that when cancer appears in a second organ, it may be a totally separate manifestation unconnected to the first, by signifying a continuing breakdown of the body's defense mechanisms. In any case, the Drs. Fishers' research has proven to all but the most recalcitrant that a surgical attack on the lymph system, no matter how extensive, has scant hope of eradicating or containing cancer.

Much of orthodoxy has had to recognize, reluctantly, that the tumor is not autonomous. The growth of the malignant cell is directly related to the conditions of the environment, principally the strength of the body's immunosuppressive system. More and more, physicians (but with few surgeons among them) are belatedly recognizing that cancer, rather than being a local affliction that will spread unless surrounded and eliminated, is a generalized or systemic disease, no doubt from its inception. That means that no local treatment is likely to have long-lasting effects on survival. Only therapy that acts throughout the body can theoretically achieve that. Despite the preponderance of evidence in this direction, the vast majority of orthodoxy has preferred to continue in entrenched error.

In 1971, an organized clinical trial to compare radical mastectomy with less extensive forms of surgical treatment was headed by Dr. Fisher, enlisting 34 U.S. and Canadian institutions and more than 1,700 patients who were assigned at random to three separate kinds of mastectomy surgery. These patients have now been followed for from six to nine years. The results have conclusively proven that there is no significant difference in longevity between patients on whom the radical surgery was perpetrated and those patients fortunate enough to receive much less severe butchery.

As a result of this test, in 1979 the NCI brought together a panel of experts to develop a consensus protocol regarding local treatment. Notice that the testing had already proven that dissimilar local treatment all still produced the same similar, dismal results — and evidense continued to pile up that cancer was systemic and not a local disease.

Still, these heads of cancer establishments failed to consider for one moment discontinuing mastectomy surgery altogether. Instead, they noted the "exciting preliminary results" and urged "continued support for such studies." Because of continuing debate between radical and conservative proponents; they still failed to endorse any less drastic surgery than has been performed for the last 90 years. Unbelievable!

Not even considered by this group was the eye-opening statistical research of Dr. Hardin Jones of the University of California. His findings indicate that those women with diagnosed breast cancer who refuse surgery stand an equal, if not better, chance of survival than patients who have been led to the operating table by their uninformed physicians and establishment-indoctrinated surgeons.

Nor did they consider the results of an autopsy study of women over 70 who died of causes other than cancer. The percentage of those women with microscopically-diagnosable breast cancer was 19 times greater than the actual incidence of overt breast cancer in that age group — conclusive evidence that these women had immuno-suppressive systems capable of handling cancer without the surgeon's knife or the radiologist's gun, although they were candidates for, and would no doubt have been victims of, these procedures had the disease been diagnosed in their lifetimes.

The evidence continues to come in from clinical testing by such internationally respected researchers as Drs. Veronesi of Italy, M. Olevski of Helsinki, Finland, and R. Calle, Foundation Curie, Paris. No matter how much or how little surgery is performed, statistically the resulting patient longevity is always the same.

We are not considering here the possible cosmetic benefits of surgery — only longevity — and certainly quality of life that is devastatingly affected both physically and psychologically by these drastic local procedures against a systemic disease of the whole body.

The butchery continues. Surgeons continue to classify their patients into Groups I, II, III, depending upon size of tumor, and debate among themselves which type of operation should be performed — radical mastectomy; modified radical mastectomy; total mastectomy; segmental mastectomy; wide excision; tumor excision; lumpectomy. No matter how you slice it, it's still human vivisection. And it offers no statistical evidence of increased longevity or patient well-being.

Establishment medicine has failed. It continues to callously persist in methods that generate profits at the cost of hundreds of thousands of lives every year.

The solution, for many, is too late. It may not be too late, however, for you. Prevention is the answer. Nutrition and metabolic therapy is the core of prevention.

In Chapter 13 we will outline a simple nutritional program that will maintain and build your natural defenses against cancer.

The recipes in the second half of this book are an integral part of prevention.

If you already have cancer, then nutrition alone may not be enough; the only solution is to seek medical advise from a doctor oriented to the metabolic approach. Under no circumstances should you attempt self-treatment. A preventive diet is common sense but once cancer is suspected, the only course is to see a doctor.

At this point, we wish to emphasize that we have attempted to produce a readable book, understandable to the layman as well as the medical professional. Technical terms and detailed scientific explanations of mechanisms have been excluded wherever possible.

There is nothing secret about the course of treatment followed by a doctor oriented to metabolic therapy. There may be some local differences due to harrassment by the police power of the state and medical orthodoxy, which finds the profits in surgery and drug dealing too great to allow quick and easy surrender to prevention or nutrition.

The logic and common sense of the protocols of preventive and metabolic medicine in cancer therapy are just as important as technical and theoretical explanations, if not more so. For the sake of easy reading, footnotes and references in this book have been kept to a minimum. Let us assure the reader that all statements contained herein have been thoroughly researched in the laboratory at Chicago's Loyola University and at equally well-equipped and respected research facilities around the world. Therapeutic evaluations and protocols are the result of work by internationally recognized medical and scientific investigators.

In addition, Dr. Manner continues to receive and computerize the clinical experience of over 150 American physicians whose subjective and empirical observations have led them to successfully practice the metabolic treatment of cancer. These physicians, who have become members of the Metabolic Research Foundation, have further joined themselves together in an association of clinics to share information on therapeutic procedures. Their regularly held seminars, workshops and reports of clinical successes continue to establish the basis for these procedures.

For those wishing to verify or pursue the scientific foundations for any of the information in this book, a complete bibliography of pertinent reference works is included. Information on the continuing research conducted in the laboratory at Loyola University or done clinically through the Metabolic Research Foundation is also available upon professional request.

The following chapter is devoted entirely to Dr. Manner's PHYSICIAN'S PROTOCOL as a guide to metabolic therapy, once the symptoms of cancer have been professionally diagnosed. It is deserving of thoughtful reading and practical application by anyone seeking an alternative to surgery.

CHAPTER 9:

The Manner Physicians Protocol

"All truth passes through three stages. First it is ridiculed; second, it is violently opposed; third, it is accepted as being self-evident."

Schoepenhauer

This guide was prepared in response to the many requests received from practicing physicians. It is presented with the full realization that modifications will undoubtedly be necessary to fit the needs of individual patients. However, this protocol should not be modified without thoughtful consideration of the consequences of deleting or substituting products.

It is with regret that the products designated herein must, of necessity, be identified by their brand, rather than generic, names. FDA regulation of these products has alternately been to ban some products from the marketplace and allow others to be distributed without matching the technical specifications for the item or meeting the standards of good pharmaceutical practice in its preparation. No therapy program can produce consistent clinical results unless the products used are consistent.

The brands mentioned here have been analyzed and used in the laboratory and clinical studies. No doubt there are other good products available. However, the purchaser would do well to remember the adage, "If you do not know what you are buying, know who you are buying it from." If you have doubt about the therapeutic efficacy of any product offered to you, it would be wise to arrange for an analysis of the product.

This protocol is solely for the practicing physician. It should in no way be considered a "do-it-yourself" therapy. Professional diagnosis and regular checkups are absolutely essential to the success of any treatment schedule.

Pre-Treatment

Without exception, the ration of minerals to other nutrients in patients exhibiting the symptons of cancer is out of balance. It is probable that selenium and zinc levels will be low. Molybdenum deficiency, which seems to be related to cancer of the esophagus, will predictably be high. Copper and lead levels are often far above average. The triglycerides and cholesterol in the blood must usually be lowered. Low manganese appears to be linked to high cholesterol levels. As the Metabolic Research Foundation, under the direction of Dr. Manner, continues to receive and computerize the laboratory reports of its member physicians, the blood and mineral profiles of homeostasis and of the potential and diagnosed cancer patient become more well defined.

A hair and blood elemental analysis should be performed to guide the physician in determining the supplementation or eliminations necessary to bring the body as close to normalcy as possible.

The laboratory norms for blood profiles represent an average for the population. As the population becomes sicker, the ranges become greater. The norms usually accompanying the standard blood tests do not represent an ideal condition from metabolic therapy's viewpoint. Dr. Manner suggested that the following ranges are more realistic.

TERMS-VALUES/TERMS-VALUES

Calcium 9.7-10.1/Potassium "serum" 4.0-4.3
Phosphorous 3.1-3.5/Chloride "serum" 100-104
Glucose 85-100/Creatinine "serum" 0.7-1.0
Bun 13-17/Iron "serum" 95-100

Uric Acid 4.5-5.5/Bun/Creatinine ratio 14.5-15.5
Cholesterol 185-215/Triglycerides 95-105
Total Protein 7.2-7.5/WBC 5000-6000
Albumen 4.0-4.4/RBC 4.5-5.0 million
Bilirubin 0.5-0.7/Hemoglobin 14.5-15.0
Alkaline Phosphatase 67.5-77.5/Hematocrit 40-50
LDH 125/135/Eosinophils 0-2
SGOT 18-22/Basophils 0-2
Total Globulin 2.8-3.5/Monocytes 4-6
A/G Ratio 2.5-3.5/Lymphocytes 34-45
Sodium "serum" 140-143/Segs 45-55

Six Methionine-200 tablets taken daily for one week should effectively remove surplus minerals. Heavy metals may take longer. Mineral supplementation will usually correct deficiencies rather quickly. As we proceed with the protocol, the diet will bring triglycerides and cholesterol to appropriate low levels.

Treatment

Phase I, First 21 Days:
1. FAST. For the first two days, patient intake must be confined strictly to fruit and vegetable juices, and the more the better. The reasons are threefold:

First, we are attempting to saturate the body with a maximum intake of full-potency, natural vitamins and minerals. It is obvious that many times the nutritional intake can be obtained by eliminating the bulk.

Second, we wish to cleanse the entire gastrointestinal system as quickly and as totally as possible, eliminating all residue toxins. We recommend adding four or five tablespoons of bran each day to the juices as an additional cleansing agent.

Third, it is essential that bowel movements become regular. At least one and preferably two to four movements a day must be achieved. The stool should become soft but well formed.

Body wastes are, themselves, carcinogenic so bowel transit time must be reduced to a minimum. Usually the increased intake of juice has a natural laxative effect. After the two-day juice fast, if frequent bowel evacuation has not been achieved, increase the amount of bran taken each day; in addition, two capsules of Lactozyme in a glass of juice taken one hour after meals should be initiated and continued until normalcy. In extreme cases it may be necessary to use colonic irrigation.

During this intial period, as much of the patient's liquid intake as is possible should be fruit and vegetable juices. When supplemental water is required, it should be pure spring water or distilled water. The chemicals in most tap water are extremely undesirable. Since various spring waters vary in mineral content, and because in some cases distilled water will chelate certain minerals from the body, the doctor should give ample consideration to the type of water recommended.

2. DETOXIFICATION. This crisis nutritional program depends upon a foundation of detoxification as complete as is possible, achieved in as short a time as possible. There is absolutely no doubt that liver dysfunction is a concommitant phenomenon of cancer. As one of the body's chief organs for the elimination and conversion of toxic substances, the livers of cancer patients have become clogged with many of the poisons they were meant to eliminate.

Dr. Buckner and Dr. Swaffield report in *Cancer Research 1973,* "100 percent of a group suffering from gastrointestinal cancer suffered liver disorder." Drs. R. Robertson and H. Kahler have reported that laboratory animals in whom they induced liver cirrhosis all developed tumors in sites as varied as lung and bladder. Cancer can be reversed and controlled only if we regenerate the liver.

Fortunately for us, the liver is the one organ in the body capable of regenerating itself. We must immediately institute a program of purification. This is helped by the natural diuretic effect of our liquid fruit and vegetable intake. In addition, the purging process will be enhanced and speeded by the daily administration of a coffee-retention enema. In cases of extreme toxemia, which is most common, these enemas should be given twice daily.

Prepare the coffee by normal percolation or drip method. *Instant coffee is not acceptable.* Preferably, the coffee should be as fresh as possible. However, it can be made and stored in the refrigerator for use within a 48-hour period. The enema should consist of a minimum 8-oz cup to the maximum of one quart at body temperature and should be retained for at least 15 to 30 minutes. The body should not be expected to accept the liquid at too fast a rate. So as to avoid cramps, the enema bag should be no higher than six inches above the bowel. Patients will find they are better able to increase both the amount and the time of the retention as they become used to the procedure.

We are fully aware of the deprecatory remarks made by the uninformed about this particular part of the detoxification process. But the importance of cleaning out the liver before commencing to rebuild the immune system cannot be over-emphasized. During the period of retention, massage the bowel and maintain a position, if possible, where the trunk of the body is higher that the head. If this is not possible, the patient should lie on the left side. It is the caffeine content of the coffee which stimulates the secretion of bile, detoxifying the liver and restoring the alkaline condition of the small intestines. Perhaps it would appear more professional to prescribe a solution of so many grains of caffeine benzoate or caffeine citrate, but coffee has proven to be the simplest and most thorough; and it is most generally available.

In addition to this daily enema, six CRP capsules should be taken daily to facilitate absorption of nutrients. If nausea occurs at any time during the treatment plan, administer six tablets daily of Cytozyme Stomach and/or Duodinal Tissue.

It is extremely important that the patient perspire heavily at least 15 minutes each day. The skin is our largest organ of excretion and, as such, acts as a third kidney in eliminating toxins from the body. Exercise is the preferable method to create the sweating condition. When this is not possible, a heat room heavy sweat clothing, or blanketing is acceptable.

3. DIGESTIVE ENZYMES. To decrease the stress placed on the gastric glands and the pancreas, one or two Hydrozyme tablets should be taken with each meal. This compound contains hydrochloric acid, pepsin and enterically-coated pancreatic enzymes. This will ensure a proper digestion of ingested foods. The patient should be given a graded litmus paper and instructed to test the first urine in the morning. It should have a pH of about 5.5. Three Trophozyme tablets daily will assist the digestive function of the small intestine. Additionally, six Cytozyme Pancreas tablets daily will help to rebuild the pancreas.

4. ENZYMES. Three Retenzyme E.C. and one Intenzyme tablet are taken together three times daily. These enzymes must be taken when the digestive tract is the most empty. They should be administered midway between breakfast and lunch, lunch and dinner, and dinner and bedtime. The 3:1 ratio must be maintained.

> NOTE: If there is a problem with oral administration of the enzyme, or if it is felt that additional enzyme therapy is required, a rectal form of the enzyme (Retenzyme Aqua +) is available. Two tablets daily are given as a retention enema.

5. VITAMIN A. This should be given in an emulsified form to prevent liver involvement. Twenty drops of Bio AE Mulsion Forte are given in morning juice and another 20 drops in the evening juice to increase the number of circulating lymphocytes. This will give the patient 500,000 IU daily. Every second day an additional 5 drops should be added morning and evening. The incidence of headache or dry, scaling skin usually indicates maximum dosage has been exceeded. When these symptoms occur, discontinue vitamin A for one week. Return after one week with a two-week on, one-week off routine, employing a 5 A.M. and 5 P.M. dosage 10 drops lower than that which caused the toxic reacion. 700,000 IU daily is the usual toxic level. Lymphocytes are activated by the addition of Cytozyme Thymus (six tablets daily).

6. VITAMIN C. Fifteen grams of ascorbic acid (or to bowel tolerance) should be given daily. This amount of ascorbic acid may cause gastric disturbances; for this reason, spread the 15 grams throughout the day. The dosage may be increased at the discretion of the physician. Some have recommended dosages as high as 50-70 grams daily. Bio C Plus (1 gram per tablet) will replace minerals while minimizing digestive upset.

Man is an exception in the animal kingdom in that he does not have the capability of manufacturing vitamin C within his own body. This is demonstrated by the case of scurvy (the sailor's calamity). When deprived of food bearing sources of this vitamin, man soon becomes ill and eventually dies. Our only source is from our food supply, which in many cases is so depleted in this previous nutrient that many of the colds, skin disorders and infirmities of modern man are actually nothing other than subclinical scurvy.

It has been laboratory proven that animals under the stress of illness increase the internal synthesis of vitamin C many-fold and supplement even this with increased intake from external sources. No doubt you have watched pet dogs and cats chew on leaves or grasses — which are not part of their normal diet — when they become sick.

Similarly, man must increase his intake of vitamin C during periods of stress. Those normal amounts of the vitamin required during periods of good health must be dramatically increased; the body itself will determine at what level, by the bowel tolerance mechanism explicated in a previous section on vitamin C.

7. VITAMIN B15. The salts of pangamic acid will increase the efficiency of cellular oxidation. Organic-15 is available as the zinc and magnesium pangamates. Two of the B15 tablets should be given with each meal or six per day.

8. AMYGDALIN. The crown jewel in this metabolic program of cancer management is the amygdalin. We have, it is hoped, balanced the body chemistry, stimulated and supplemented the immune system with enzymes that will seek out and destroy the protective protein coat surrounding the cancer cell, reduced toxemia, oxygenated the blood, and cleansed the liver.

Now we supply the extrinsic amygdalin that helps our body destroy the cancer cell by the mechanism explained previously.

Four choices of administration are open to the physician, depending upon such factors as patient condition, progress of the disease, location and ancillary treatments, if any. These are medical decisions that vary greatly with each patient and the medical philosophy of the doctor. We suggest that the inexperienced physician accept consultation when making the decision on route of administration. Many times, a combination of systems is advisable.

Intravenous: Three 3-gram vials injected — IV push. A subjective response should be noted within 48 hours (increased appetite, lower blood pressure, increased feeling of well-being, release from pain). If this response is not noted, increase the injection by 3 grams each day up to 30 grams or until a definite positive response is achieved. When administered in the large amounts, the amygdalin should be placed in a physiological solution and injected within 20 to 30 minutes.

According to Dr. E. T. Krebs, if you have the real natural laevo material the amount can be excessive only in economic terms. There is hope that the future holds the promise of higher dosages obtainable at reduced capital outlay. Dr. Krebs has pointed to the extremely high L.D. of amygdalin. In rabbits it has been shown to be 20,000 mg/kg IV. We can only speculate that the L.D. is so high, and amygdalin so nontoxic, because it is inherent within the human biological experience. Based on the above information we can theorize that in a 150-lb. man, lethal toxicity would occur at a level of approximately 1200 gm IV. When we analyze the successful animal studies which have been done with amygdalin, we find dosage levels of 500, 1000, 1500, and 2000 mg/kg of body weight having been employed. If we equate a medium range dose of 1000 mg/kg to a 150-lb. man we find the parenteral dose to be approximately 60 grams. Even if we take into consideration the lesser efficiency of an intramuscular (IM) injection in mice vs. IV in humans, we still must assume a level of efficacy at somewhere between 30 to 60 grams.

As stated previously, only amygdalin packaged in its crystalline form and dissolved in sterile water just prior to use has proven satisfactory for intravenous injection. The use of preparations packed in liquid form is definitely not recommended. Clinical and laboratory tests of the brand Laevalin has consistently shown it to be full-potency, natural amygdalin.

Oral: Therapeutic efficacy of amygdalin is considered by many authorities to be highest when the natural metabolic pathway of oral ingestion is followed. Tablets are, therefore, the delivery system recommended by the majority of physicians when the patient's digestive system is still functioning normally. Six 500 mg Laevalin tablets (2 TID) should be taken daily by mouth (3 grams), specifically at meal times. Some patients say they experience a slight nausea or stomach distress. A small amount of Maalox or Milk of Magnesia will usually eliminate this. Once again, subjective improvement should be noticed within a short period. Some doctors regularly prescribe considerably larger amounts. The patient should be carefully monitored to determine tolerance level.

Inasmuch as present law requires that most amygdalin be extracted abroad, it is not subject to FDA purview. Many of the tablets in circulation have been sub-strength. Some that we have tested contained no amygdalin at all.

Special care must be taken that the tablets used contain only natural laevo amygdalin in the amount specified. Tablets should be identified by the trademark of their manufacturer, who should be willing to include or send a thorough analysis of his product by an independent United States laboratory. Our recommendation of Laevalin is based upon having continually found this tablet to maintain excellent pharmaceutical standards.

Rectal: Place one 3-gram vial of Laevalin, or crush six 500 mg tablets in 50-100 cc of warm tap water. Agitate until fully dissolved. Using a 100-cc syringe with plastic tube attached, insert into the rectum.

This procedure should be commenced only after completion of the coffee enema. The liquid should then be retained until the next bowel movement. This compromise method of administration offers the advantages of the IV administration in that the amygdalin is quickly absorbed into the bloodstream via the portal vein directly to the liver. There is no gastrointestinal distress and usually higher amounts may be taken than with the oral delivery method. This rectal method also offers the advantages of the oral in that the enzymatic breakdown of the amygdalin is easily accomplished in the bowel. Those patients who either fear the needle or have poor vein structure can avoid the trauma of injection but still receive quick assimilation into the blood.

The disadvantage may be in an extremely high amount of betaglucosidase contained in fecal matter retained in the lower intestines. Such high concentration could precipitate too extensive an enzymatic conversion of the amygdalin resulting in a toxic reaction and must, therefore, be closely monitored by the physician. When administration is made after the regular coffee enema the process should be safe and results have been excellent. This method is often combined with oral administration of Laevalin tablets.

Intramuscular Injection: Dr. Davis at American Hospital in Zion, Illinois, has reported results by IM or subcutaneous injection which he feels equal those given intravenously. He reports the subcutaneous absorption is complete in approximately 30 minutes.

9. VITAMIN MINERAL SUPPLEMENT. A therapeutic vitamin-mineral preparation such as Multidyn should be given morning and evening, or four per day.

10. OTHER SUPPLEMENTS. Other nutritional supplements can be considered for individual cases. Selenium, zinc, RNA-DNA and vitamin E have been used with excellent therapeutic effects. There is no supplement which cannot be taken safetly with the aforementioned plan. In fact, one should supplement 12 tablets daily of the gland or organ tissue primarily affected. Most patients are hypoglycemic, so the adrenals, thyroid and liver should be supplemented. Six tablets each daily of Cytozyme Adrenal, Cytozyme Thyroid and Cytozyme Liver should be

taken. If there is a past history of radiation and/or chemotherapy, Dismuzyme is recommended (six tablets per day).

11. DIET. This is the most important component of the treatment because it involves a change in lifestyle and eating habits. The recipes in the second section, it is hoped, will show that this diet, once past the initial phase, need not be unappetizing. In the beginning, strict adherence must be maintained. The slightest deviance may prevent the body from reaching homeostasis and result in failure for the entire metabolic therapy.

A juice extractor should be purchased, and most of the vegetables in the diet juiced in this way so that all of the naturally-occurring enzymes, minerals and vitamins will be present. These fresh juices may be warmed slightly to make a soup, but never heat beyond 107°F, the point at which the enzymes will be destroyed. At least 64 ounces of raw juice each day should be consumed.

We would like to maintain a good fiber content in the system, obtainable in bran as well as in whole, raw vegetables. The amount will be determined, of course, by the physician, depending upon the location of the tumor. Other variables will be determined by individual situations and the effects of additional diseases such as diabetes, hypoglycemia, arteriosclerosis, heart problems and allergies.

I recently had the sad experience of calling on an acquaintance who had been diagnosed as terminally ill with cancer. Visiting with him was one of his personal friends, who happens to be one of the most respected and most orthodox physicians in our community. This doctor had doubtless been exposed to less than a four-hour course in nutrition during his entire medical education — and his wife, through kitchen experience, was probably better qualified to give nutritional information. Yet here was my friend being advised by this ill-informed doctor to build his resistance with increased protein intake of good red meat — and to maintain his body weight and energy by drinking milkshakes! Such misguided and presumptuous recommendations are repeated regularly by doctors whose ignorance of the epidemiological link to cancer of these foundations of the American diet continues to jeopardize the health of their patients.

The rationale of diet in the prevention of cancer will be more thoroughly explicated in the following chapter. Suffice it to say here that in crisis situations where cancer symptoms have become manifest, we *must* have a crisis diet.

Fats must be reduced to an absolute minimum in order to reduce levels in the blood stream of triglycerides and fatty globules, both of which inhibit oxygen transference to the cells. And cholesterol must be *totally* eliminated in order to ease liver function. (Dr. R. Steiner, in *Cancer Research 1942,* noted that cholesterol alone was capable of inducing tumors in mice; in humans, impaired cholesterol metabolism is a common cause of cancers, since oleic acid leads to fatty liver generation.) Animal proteins will be totally eliminated from the diet to allow the bowel to establish the proper flora for the generation of beta-glucosidase, which commences the breakdown processes of amygdalin in the nitriloside foods that will be included in the nutritional mix, and also reduce digestive need for the pancreatic enzymes. Sugar, caffeine and salt, all of which have been linked to carcinogenic metabolic process within the body, must be eliminated throughout the first three-week program.

The diet will consist almost exclusively of unrefined carbohydrates. This is a *crisis diet* for a *crisis situation.* It must be maintained with no exceptions. Not only is it the foundation for immediate reversal of cancer metabolism, but at the end of the three-week period the patient is going to find that his desire for foods that are toxic, carcinogenic and otherwise metabolically inappropriate has completely disappeared. Moreover, the patient will easily accept the dietary habits that will be necessary to reinforce and support the immune system for the rest of his life.

Patients on this diet should not lose weight, other than that which is excessive for their height and bone structure. This is extremely desirable. The physician, if he feels the weight loss is excessive, should prescribe two to four tablets of free form amino acids taken daily; this will supply amino acids which do not require pancreatic enzymes for body assimilation.

In the past, we have been reluctant to recommend any of the predigested proteins due to the inconsistencies in their manufacture, and to the high incidence of allergic reaction and loss of bone density during their use. But the recent introduction of free amino acids has been found to overcome these objections and they are recommended where necessary.

Category	Foods Allowed	Foods to Avoid
Beverages	Herb teas; fresh fruit juices; fresh vegetable juice	Alcohol; cocoa; coffee; carbonated and canned drinks; artificial fruit drinks; regular tea
Dairy Products	Raw, skim or non-fat milk on cereal only; non-fat yogurt; non-fat cottage cheese; whole milk and/or cream for sauces only in limited amounts	Butter; margarine; ice cream
Eggs	Egg whites only	No whole eggs in any form
Fish	None (during first three weeks)	All
Fruits	All - fresh, dried, un-sulphured; frozen; un-sweetened, whole when possible, including seeds or kernels	Canned; sweetened; avocado
Grains	All whole-grain cereals; millet; buckwheat; oats; rye; wheat; breads made from these without sugar and eggs	Processed grains, such as white rice; refined wheat; crackers, including bran; macaroni; prepared cereals; pita bread (if refined flour)
Nuts	All nuts and seeds, pre-ferably raw; dry-roasted, if necessary; sunflower; soy nuts; pumpkin	Roasted in oil; salted peanuts

Oils	None	Shortening; refined oil, both saturated and unsaturated; margarine; olive oil
Seasonings	Herbs; garlic salt; onion; thyme; cayenne; parsley; marjoram; basil; celery salt; soy sauce; preservative-free salza; wine flavoring only; seeds; raisins	Salt
Soup	All made from scratch in blender, salt-free; asparagus; bean; tomato; millet	Canned; creamed; bouillon
Sprouts	All, especially millet, soy, lentil, alfalfa, mung	Potato, Tomato
Sweeteners	Frozen fruit concentrates containing no sugar; raisins	Honey; refined sugar, white or brown; syrups
Vegetables	All, cooked as little as possible, preferably not over 107°F. (Clean all vegetables thoroughly to eliminate surface contaminants. All beverage and food preparation must be done with only pure bottled water in stainless steel, ceramic or glass utensils. There can be no exceptions	All canned, prepared

For the individual who resists a diet regimen as strict as we outline, let us emphasize again this is a *crisis diet* for only a three-week period. We are attempting to overcome the overt symptoms of a killer disease that has been preparing its assault on the body for as long as 15 years. The alternative is an early and possibly agonizing demise.

For clarity, this is not strictly a salt-free diet, as we include celery salt, soya, and preservative-free salzas. The imaginative cook can make many combinations of tasty herb, yogurt, and cottage cheese sauces for combined vegetable dishes and add texture with seeds and sprouts. Only fructose sugar is sparingly allowed. Sugar-free fruit concentrate on pita bread or whole-grain muffins are really delicious. Salad dressing of salza and herbs can be quite appetizing. Remember, this isn't forever. What is three weeks compared to a lifetime?

Additional Ancillary Therapy

The principal causes of cancer death, although nonexclusive and overlapping, are:

1. Mechanical interference with the function of a vital organ.
2. Toxemia.
3. Side effects of chemotherapy and radiation.
4. The depression or destruction of the immune system, allowing an additional chronic or viral disease to invade the body and provide the final *coup de grace.*
5. Dysfunction of the psyche.
6. Cachexia — the gradual wasting away of the body. The patient becomes mentally listless, physically without energy, and this condition is accompanied by a rapid loss of weight.

Cancerous tumor cells derive their energy for growth and division from the fermentation of glucose. The malignant cell requires more than 50 times more glucose than a normal cell. This glucose is fermented into lactic acid which returns by way of the blood stream to the liver and kidneys where it is recycled back to glucose. This process, called gluconeogenesis (gluco-neo-genesis), consumes body energy and is an extremely wasteful metabolism that causes the breakdown of tissue proteins into their amino acids, which are then converted into the glucose the tumor demands for fuel. The tumor grows at the expense of deteriorating muscle and connective tissue throughout the body, which self-destructively degenerates away. This is classic cachexia.

Amygdalin normally increases patient appetite to deter cachexia; the diet is designed to stabilize and reverse this process by increasing blood oxygenation and limiting fermentation.

In cases where the patient comes to the physician in an advanced state of cachexatic deterioration and continues to sink into malaise, immediate therapeutic effects have been achieved by the administration of hydrazine sulfate, which appears to block this devastating metabolism.

Considerable research into the process of gluconeogenesis has been done by Joseph Gold, M.D., of Syracuse University, and Dean Burke, Ph.D., formerly with National Cancer Institute, both of whom find this therapy extremely beneficial.

Hydrazine sulfate should be taken on an empty stomach, before dinner, lunch, or bedtime. For a person 130 lbs. or over, two 60-mg capsules — one taken in the morning and one at night — is the usual physician-prescribed amount. For a person less than this weight, 30-mg tablets on the same schedule should prove sufficient.

Some doctors recommend dietary inclusion of natural yogurt or acidophilus capsules to seed the intestines with the betaglucosidase necessary for the first enzymatic breakdown of amygdalin. Betaglucosidase is an excretion product of the acidophilus bacilli. Many times these acid bacilli will not be contained in sufficient quantity in the intestine where meat is the principal ingested food. Our diet of unrefined carbohydrates provides the environment for proper bacterial concentration, so additional sources of acidophilus, while welcome, should not be necessary.

The precursors of cancer include maladaption to stress, mental as well as physical. Biofeedback, Bible study, anything leading to a relaxed mental attitude, have all proven helpful. To the greatest extent possible, the patient's family and friends should be totally supportive and remove as much stress and turmoil from the environment as they can. A patient's good mental attitude is part of the protocol every physician would like to prescribe. Unfortunately, it must originate within the patient himself.

The experience of metabolic physicians is conclusive that patients who say, "Doctor, show me how to heal myself," have far better chances for survival than those patients who expect the doctor, alone, to provide a miracle. The fighters survive. They stick to the diet. They remain faithful to their medication. And their positive attitude provides the climate for self healing. Every possible avenue should be taken to develop in the patient the proper psyche for self healing.

It should be unnecessary to state that all carcinogenic substances or environments should be avoided. No smoking. Avoid smog or congested streets and areas whenever possible. Food selected should be as organically raised as possible, without pesticides and preservatives.

The protocol outlined here for a crisis situation is not designed to fight only an invasive condition, as orthodoxy attempts to do with its radiation, drugs and surgery directed against the lump or bump. Metabolic physicians recognize that these symptoms are just the *final* result of an underlying metabolic imbalance and weakened immune system.

CHAPTER 10:

Biological Experience and Cancer Prevention

"Our present system recognizes disease only when it has reached crisis proportions. This is tantamount to saying that a fire is only a fire when it has burst through the roof when, in actuality, it was a fire when the cigarette butt began to smolder in the rug."

Carlton Frederics

Cancer, like most diseases, is preceded by a latency period until its symptoms may no longer be ignored. Cancer does not start with a tumor. The tumor is simply the irreversible symptom. It is known that a chest tumor becomes visible on X-ray only after its diameter has reached five to 10mm.

Katakowski and Gerstenberg proved conclusively that some tumors require at least 15 years to grow from the first fermenting cell to cell masses in diagnosable form. The latency period of cancer has been estimated to be four times longer than its diagnosable or clinical stage. Only when the tumor becomes obvious and recognized does orthodox medicine commence its crisis treatment of surgery, poisoning or burning.

The established medical community continually warns to avoid one substance or environment after another. Almost every day our newspapers present yet another cancer irritant exposed by the FDA, the NCI or the ACS. One tongue-in-cheek story circulated recently about these stalwart guardians of our health is that they have now determined that saliva is a cause of cancer when swallowed in small amounts over a prolonged period of time.

All we are offered, after billions of tax and contributed research dollars, are negative solutions — things to avoid, like environments, food additives, smoking and a continually lengthening list of carcinogens. But never one positive action that we can take by way of preparing our bodies to prevent cancer, or to provide immunity to contact with these substances — which, in truth, only trigger the cancer or determine the location in which it will strike, as no doubt cigarettes do in the case of lung cancer.

The cancer establishment (the whole alphabet of governmental and contribution-supported agencies) professes to see light at the end of the tunnel. Yet all the while they admit that they haven't yet found the cause of cancer. As a consequence, no positive program has ever been presented to enable Americans to prepare their bodies to prevent the onslaught of the dread disease. Most often, the light at the end of the tunnel is, for the afflicted, an incinerator or, as some suggest, "an oncoming train."

Immunity Through Biological Experience

The holistic- or metabolically-oriented physician recognizes the natural intrinsic immune system designed into the human body and the extrinsic backup system provided in our natural food supply. Basically, the natural resistance of the body to disease must be maintained and any inherited weakness of the natural immune system within our body strengthened or overcome. How? Simply by returning to our bodies the food substances natural to man's biological experience and eliminating non-foods that place unanticipated stresses on our metabolic systems.

As exhibited in all chronic metabolic diseases — scurvy, pellagra, etc. — the final resolution has always been found to be nutritional, and the prevention always the same as the cure.

At many medical symposiums at which I have lectured I have asked the audience to name one chronic metabolic disease where the eventual control was not found to be dietary. I have never been challenged. Cancer is no exception.

In the previous chapter a model, but not definitive, protocol was presented for the patient to whom the knowledge of prevention has come too late. It will be noted that after detoxification of the body, the treatment consists principally of attempting to rebuild its metabolic balance or homeostasis with vitamins, minerals and enzymes, the goal of which is to reactivate the immune system for a massive resistance to the already entrenched enemy. How much better it would be if the body's forces of resistance had been nurtured and maintained throughout life!

The bad news as provided by American Cancer Society statistics is that one out of every four Americans alive today will contract cancer. The good news is that by following a very simple nutritional program you will never be that one and you are going to feel better and live better than ever before.

Simply stated, the cancer prevention diet in this chapter acts to return your body to the nutritional environment it was originally designed for.

Every fine piece of machinery leaves the factory with included directions for care and maintenance, as specified by its designers. Your automobile, for instance, is delivered with a maintenance manual that specifies the octane rating of gasoline to be used, the viscosity of the lubricating oil, the weight of transmission fluid, the type of air cleaner and oil filter, the grade of coolant required in the radiator. Your automobile will operate at maximum efficiency and last longer if you use the lubricants and fuels specified.

It has been suggested that the many references to nutrition in the Bible, beginning with Genesis 1:29, could be considered the maintenance book from our designer and manufacturer. Certainly, the Biblical references to diet are exacting and correlate to the cancer prevention program we recommend.

The human body is an intricately designed and balanced machine. Each metabolic system within the whole is integrated and matched for the total life-support mechanism. When all systems are functioning properly, the body is remarkably resilient to trauma. Like any other fine piece of machinery, the body has safety margins and tolerance included in its design which allow it to temporarily continue functioning even though not fueled properly.

Referring again to our analogous automobile, while all fuels and lubricants have been definitively specified, the machinery can tolerate, for limited periods, low-octane gasoline, impure air and contaminated lubricants. The machinery will continue to operate. Built into the machinery are safety factors that allow the equipment to function above or below factory specified norms. In addition, the engine is equipped with various filters and cleaners which eliminate many harmful contaminants.

Eventually, however, improper maintenance will have its deleterious effect. Perhaps starting will be a little difficult, pick-up will be sluggish, vibration will occur in idle, or there may be a cloudy exhaust. Some or all of these minor symptoms of inadequate lubrication and fueling will sooner or later appear. Though these symptoms are irritating, the automobile will still continue to provide transportation. At this stage, returning the machine to optimum performance can be accomplished by resuming the use of proper fuels and lubricants. The alternative is eventual major breakdowns, staggering repair bills and, finally, total loss of function.

Similarly, the human body has intrinsic protective mechanisms and tolerance factors that allow it to continue to function under abusive conditions. Modern man fuels his body, more often than not, with inadequate, improper nutrition that does not meet the design specifications of his Creator for the prevention of degenerative disease.

The human race was placed in a totally integrated environment so perfectly designed that it could not have just happened. That man has taken this biological heritage, so perfectly designed for his needs, and perverted, separated and converted its basic nutritional elements is the major causative factor of degenerative disease.

The maintenance of your body's defense against all degenerative disease — and these include arteriosclerosis, arthritis, heart disease, etc. — depends upon returning to the nutrition of our inherited biological experience. We will, henceforth, refer to the Bio-X Diet as that nutritional program that includes all of the balanced food of our biological experience.

Much remains to be learned about nutrition, but within the realm of knowledge so far exposed to us we hope to show you how this diet makes scientific and common sense in its naturalness.

Information on Cancer Nutrition Limited

During the last decade we have seen numerous books published on health maintenance diets. We are not referring to the never-ending stream of fat-reducing fad diets and various other types, such as those for the Drinking Man, people who do not wish to count calories, people who are content to exist solely on protein or cellulose, and so on. These diets are too numerous, and most of them too silly — and even dangerous — to discuss seriously. There is, however, an increasing number of qualified doctors and scientists who recognize what should be patently obvious to the entire medical community. These men, all experts in their own fields, have written diet programs for the prevention of one or more of the degenerative diseases, many of which provide excellent advice. Almost without exception, these books and papers have skirted the issue of cancer. In some cases, it is because the authors still cling to the remnant of their education that dictated a belief in the microbe and localized situs theory of cancer. Perhaps it is because their scientific effort was concentrated in, and confined to, their own specialty without concern for the effects of their proposed diets on the prevention of malignancy. Possibly it is the fact that the medical/industrial/governmental complex has succeeded, without fail, in destroying the careers of capable scientists who dared to challenge the orthodox treatment of cancer by suggesting a nutritional solution. These include such eminently-qualified and respected scientists as Hoxey, Gerson and Ivy.

Without exception, all of the diets so far proposed for the prevention of any degenerative disease require the elimination of certain foods from the diet, i.e. meat, sugar, eggs, and so on. Little search has been made for foods that may have been previously removed from our food intake, thereby eliminating a possible extrinsic protective mechanism required for health maintenance, and should be returned to our diet.

While the Bio-X Diet is an excellent one for all degenerative diseases, including aging, our explanatory efforts will concentrate particularly on cancer and what should specifically be included in the food intake and what should be moderated to prevent malignancy. We know of no degenerative disease for which the Bio-X Diet is contraindicated or, indeed, is not an excellent nutritional program.

The simple rule of thumb that will henceforth guide us to maintain a cancer-free body is EAT AS CLOSE TO THE BIOLOGICAL EXPERIENCE OF OUR PREHISTORIC FOREFATHERS AS IS POSSIBLE IN A MODERN WORLD. As you will see, this requires more common sense than asceticism.

So far as we have been able to discern, there has been no discovered incidence of cancer among any wild animals killed in the hunt; yet these same species, when domesticated or placed in zoos where they must eat the foods prepared for them by man, suffer from the same epidemiological cancer found in homo sapiens. The foods prepared by their keepers might be nutritional in most respects. But they fail to contain those unrecognized, cancer-protective nutrients available intrinsically in their natural food chain. The cultivated carbohydrates and the domesticated meat products available for animal feeds, as an example, are not rich in the nitrilosides available to these animals in their natural habitats. This simple empirical observation alone should have stimulated the investigation of nutrition as it affects the incidence of cancer.

Until recently, those few in the medical profession who exhibited interest in the preventive aspect of good nutrition were thwarted in attempting to find a thoroughly non-prejudiced source of education. Medical schools, until the present, have included no required courses in nutrition in their curricula. The U.S. Health & Human Services Department is a captive of producer organizations and lobbies, each competing for a larger share of the consumer dollar with such slogans as: "Everybody Needs Milk", "Sugar, The Quick Energy Food", "Meat, The Complete Protein." Agriculture is the cornerstone of our nation's economy. We cannot expect education from our government that might reflect negatively on some section of this national resource.

We recently had the opportunity to examine the course catalogue of two of the nation's major agricultural colleges. Not one course in human nutrition was available, although a large portion of the education in animal husbandry was concerned with the feeding of domesticated animals. By contrast, schools of veterinary medicine recognize the value of nutrition in animal health maintenance. The importance of this area of veterinary education is exhibited during each visit with your dog or cat to a small-animal clinic. Invariably, the doctor will ask, "What have you been feeding this animal?" We sincerely doubt that your personal physician has ever considered your diet as a primary cause of any symptom, other than acne or stomach-ache. Certainly his medical school never trained him to do so.

Foods Themselves Are Being Changed

The scientific study of animal nutrition is researched not only in our large agricultural universities, but also by such giant food conglomerates as Ralston Purina and General Foods. These companies maintain experimental flocks and herds of meat animals which include control groups under constant study to determine methods of hastening reproduction, accelerating growth rate, and achieving higher production of butterfat, eggs and other farm products through variation in feed and chemical supplementation. Animals are selectively bred to produce progeny that reach market earlier or in a more advanced state of maturation.

Since the days of Luther Burbank, horticultural experts have hybridized our food supply until many of our grains cannot even reproduce themselves. All efforts are bent at increased yield per acre and earlier ripening. The tomatoes, corn, wheat and rice of the present era bear scant resemblance to their original conformation. If the resultant crops of this artificial selection and cultivation system provide a higher or more complete nutrition, it is purely by accident. Usually the opposite is true. The desire for earlier maturity in both animals and plants has resulted in diminished nutritional value.

The introduction of chemical fertilizers and pesticides is an additional factor that has not only resulted in lower natural nutritive quality but has introduced substances that are, indeed, dietarily harmful. The succulent flavor and satisfying appearance of home-grown vegetables is often the result of a most fortunate ignorance on the part of a gardener, unindoctrinated in the various harmful chemicals available, who is satisfied with the naturally-selected and ripened harvest provided by a more natural horticulture.

Our government tells us that half of the world presently exists on a deficient food supply. Does it not it seem logical, then, that some of these minimum-subsistence populations (already supported with food shipped by the generosity and concern of the United States) might serve as ideal experimental and control groups for the determination of human nutritional needs and solutions to nutritional problems that cannot be found through research on laboratory animals? Such research would not take advantage of an impoverished people, but would be conducted to predetermine and program the real nutritional requirements for future generations of stronger, more disease-resistant societies.

Unfortunately, the continuing nutritional research in animal husbandry does not extend to the selection and development of proper nutritional plants and animals for human consumption, only for progressively earlier production of those plants and animals. Our United States Departments of Health or Agriculture have never proposed or underwritten such basic nutritional research in the available world laboratory. This fact, we believe, indicates their lack of desire to support studies that might suggest that some of our agricultural production at home is nutritionally unsound.

Agricultural science continues its efforts to transform our natural food supply by developing produce that will be the right size to can or pick mechanically, that will be more resistant to storage and shipping damage, that will be the proper packaging size — almost always resulting in reduced food values in the hybridized product. These nutritional changes, like it or not, have been the unfortunate aftermath of the mechanization and urbanization of modern Euro-American civilization.

Cancer, A Disease of Civilization

Mark Twain wrote that man was the only animal that eats when he is not hungry and makes love in all seasons. We will not speculate on the latter. But certainly the social evolution of man, from the cave to the high-rise apartment, has seen changes that not only dictate, but in some cases require, a change in eating habit as well as in nutritional requirements.

Cancer has been called a disease of civilization. The more primitive a society and simpler its diet, the less its incidence of cancer. W. A. Price, D.D.S., author of the classic book, *Nutrition and Physical Degeneration,* crossed five continents without finding evidence of cancer in isolated self-sufficient societies. American medical teams in isolated areas of Ecuador and Brazil, studying over 60,000 inhabitants, report no know cases of cancer. Dr. S. Benet found no cancer among the Abkhasians and Hunza. Dr. Namalas F. Yaj states Australian aborigines in native environment have no cancer symptoms. At his African medical clinic, Dr. Albert E. Schweitzer stated that where there was no civilization, there was no cancer.

Aboriginal man was non-agrarian. Life was a constant search for food which could not be preserved or stored. The most physical type of modern employment would be considered sedentary compared to the caloric energy expended by our ancestral forebears just to remain warm. Many foods were available only seasonally. Life was literally feast and famine, with the latter probably predominant. All foods were eaten whole, raw, when available, at irregular intervals, and seldom mixed with other varieties. Defecation was at the immediate call of nature.

Thousands of years later, the descendant of ancient man dresses warmly in the morning. After a breakfast of prepackaged food he rides to a heated or air-conditioned office or factory. At noon the eating ritual is performed again with a mixed variety of non-food items. Afternoons are sustained with the help of artificially-created beverages. Bowel movements are scheduled for convenience, not necessity, often being delayed for long periods. Afternoons end with an air-conditioned return to one's home and, again, the eating ceremony where foods — created unnaturally, raised artificially, and heated to destruction — are mixed in abundance to please the palate rather than the nutritional demands of the body.

Our modern man has, indeed, lived his day to eat. His ancestor was hoping to eat enough just to live. The American medical profession thrives on the product of civilized eating habits which are undeniably epidemiologically responsible for a host of degenerative diseases. While orthodoxy sometimes grudgingly admits some merit in nutrition as both prevention and a solution to the problem of degeneration, it does not see it as profit. We need look no further than the political pressure exerted to make vitamins a prescription item and limit their quantitative use to determine the motives of the United States drug industry. The previously mentioned absence of nutritional education in medical schools is indicative of orthodox medicine's lack of interest.

It has been left to a few pioneer nutritionists to research and publish, for both the professional and the layman, specific dietary recommendations for degenerative disease. These diets have been given various titles: The Low-Cholesterol Diet, The Live Longer Now Diet, the LaCosta Diet, the Body Awareness Diet, the S.G.A. Diet. All of them have merit. All have a common direction: to balance nutritional intake, reduce fat and sugar, and cut down on red meat. Many of these diets receive wide circulation and are even grudgingly accepted in areas of orthodoxy as inclusive treatment for arthritis, arteriosclerosis and heart problems. Cancer is seldom mentioned in these works, since to do so would be to threaten the very foundation of medical practice and render the balance of the dietary theory unacceptable quackery.

What We Don't Eat Causes Cancer

Nutritional authors regularly cite research that tends to prove that whenever man, because of deprivation, geographical necessity or cultural preferences, exists on a diet high in one particular type of food the result is degenerative disease. The researchers follow a progression of logic that leads to a simplistic conclusion: excessive food is the causative factor of disease. Seldom do they consider that what is *left out* of the diet may be the true culprit. In the few cases where cancer is mentioned in passing, by these authorities, it is usually to cite populations of heavy meat or fat eaters as having high incidences of cancer. One would almost surmise that these authors have selected research that fits a preconceived premise.

The fact is that the various cultures that exhibit the lowest cancer rates can have varied dietary habits and preferences. It is true, for example, that those cultures with the consistently lowest cancer rates are mainly vegetarian and nutritionally oriented to diets high in complex carbohydrates — yet in cultures like the Northern Eskimo, with negligible vegetable intake and a cultural preference for blubber and similar animal fats, cancer is virtually unknown. Or take the Bantu or Masai of Africa, whose diet is almost exclusively red meat or blood and milk — these natives are also cancer-free. The one thing common to all diets of cancer-free cultures is the inclusion of nitrilosides that are contained in amounts over 500 times the daily inclusion in the diets of modern Europeans and Americans.

In the case of the Eskimo, large residual amounts of nitrilosides (amygdalin) are obtained from the staple meat of the caribou that feeds itself on the nitriloside-rich salmon berries abundant in northern latitudes. African tribesmen commonly consider the rumen contents (first stomach) of grazing animals a delicacy. These animals regularly forage on plants of extremely high nitriloside content.

With these diverse cultural eating patterns being cancer-free, logic concludes it is not what we eat but what we do *not* eat that results in cancer. Incidentally, it should be pointed out that while the aforementioned Eskimos, Bantu and Masai have no cancer because of their high intake of nitrilosides, they do suffer the extremely high incidence of other degenerative diseases you would expect from high-fat meat diets. This is, in itself, indicative of the specific extrinsic cancer prevention we receive by including nitriloside-containing plants in our diet. No matter how otherwise unhealthful a diet is, the inclusion of high-nitriloside, amygdalin content seems to prevent the incidence of cancer.

The Bio-X Diet restores to the American diet the nitriloside foods that our modern culture, agricultural economy, and eating habits have virtually eliminated over the last 50 years.

The United States Department of Agriculture Fitness Diet

Leaflet 424, revised 1964, of the USDA is entitled, "Food For Fitness," and presents a daily food guide based upon the four popular food groups: Vegetables and Fruit, Milk, Meat, Bread and Grains. The guide's daily recommendation for adults is four or more servings of vegetable and fruit, two or more servings of meat, two cups of milk and four or more servings of grain products, including refined grains. To round out this melange, the USDA in recent years has recommended two more food groups or items which they state add additional food energy and food value, but are not included in the four basic categories. These items are fats (butter, cooking oil, mayonnaise) and sugar (in and on everything). It is interesting to note the recommended percentages of carbohydrates, protein and fat in a list of foods in keeping with the USDA Daily Food Guide:

The following food mix is in keeping with the USDA Daily Food Guide (The Fitness Diet):

	PROTEIN 100			CARBOHYDRATES 100			FAT 100		
	Calories	Grams	%	Calories	Grams	%	Calories	Grams	%
Meat (including eggs)	740	47.9	61.2	--	--	--	--	58.5	39.9
Milk	322	16.6	21.4	--	23.6	9.3	--	18.0	12.2
Fruit & Vegetables	225	6.3	8.1	--	52.1	20.6	--	.9	.6
Grains (including refined)	248	6.7	8.6	--	35.8	14.1	--	1.0	.6
Sugar (5 oz.)	547	--	--	--	141.0	55.8	--	--	--
Fats (Butter, etc.)	610	--	--	--	--	--	--	68.0	46.4
Totals:	2692	77.5	100.0	--	252.5	100.0	--	146.4	100.0

Total Grams Nutrition: 16% Protein; 53% Carbohydrates; 31% Fat
Total Calories: 49% Fat; 20% Refined Sugar and Sucrose

It has been said that a giraffe is a horse that was designed by a bureaucrat. This diet is a political program designed by the USDA to provide each segment of our Agricultural Industry its fair and equal share of the food dollar. Little scientific thought about nutrition has ever been entertained by the Department of Agriculture that would change this agricultural status quo (or, incidentally, reduce its multimillion-dollar subsidy to tobacco agriculture). To do so would be to bring down the intense political pressure by a lobby each of the major agricultural producers maintains in Washington. What bureaucrat wants that?

The USDA Fitness Diet has been propagated and recommended to the American people through four decades of governmental propaganda. This is a diet designed by bureaucrats to please the politicians of each agricultural area. We challenge the USDA to find a single knowledgeable nutritionist who will not writhe in anguish at such a program. Ezra Taft Benson, former Secretary of Agriculture, resigned his position in midterm, giving as his reason that the USDA was riddled with administrative incompetents and political advocates interested only in ending our republican form of government. Such incompetency and misdirection of purpose still evidences itself in the continued propagation of this nutritionally-disastrous fitness diet.

As stated previously, we know of no contraindications for the Bio-X Diet other than, of course, specific cases of allergy, diabetes, etc. The Bio-X Diet will be beneficial for all degenerative disease but we concern ourselves here specifically with cancer and its prevention.

Comparison of USDA Fitness Diet and the Bio-X Diet

Meat:
Historically, the eating of meat in any society has been directly proportionate to its wealth and degree of civilization. The amount of cancer has also appeared in approximately the same proportions. It is this observation that has led some researchers to conclude that meat should be totally eliminated from the diet. They cite the excessive fat content of meat — the fact that the body cannot store appreciable amounts of protein, with the balance burned as energy or becoming fat. They correctly assert that high animal protein also causes inefficient elimination resulting in intestinal putrefaction and toxic buildup. The argument is cited by advocates of eliminating meat that if man were meant to be a meat eater, he would possess the much shorter intestinal system common to all carnivores.

More moderate nutritionists point out that neither does man have the extra stomachs or rumen possessed by herbivores. In truth, man possesses digestive functions of both, i.e., the grinding teeth of the herbivores and the eye or canine teeth of carnivores. By design and biological experience, man is a true omnivore with the ability of digest both meat and vegetables. Therefore, meat is definitely included in the Bio-X Diet.

There is definite merit in much of the vegetarian resistance to meat. American and European dependence upon meat as the focal point of the eating ceremony has raised the consumption of animal protein far beyond our body's ability to anticipate such excess.

The pancreatic enzymes necessary for meat digestion share a responsibility as part of the intrinsic defense against cancer. When digestive demand surpasses enzyme production capacity not only does digestion fail and allow toxemia to commence, but the immune system malfunctions.

Earliest man was protected from the possibility of continuing excesses, as he possessed neither the weapons nor the physical ability to kill the large animals of his time. Only on rare occasions when these animals were killed by accident or by their own kind, was man able to scavenge heavy meats into his diet. On these occasions the aboriginal no doubt gorged himself, to the exclusion of other foods, in the knowledge that they were so rarely available.

Of equal relevance to our biological experience is today's unnatural meat supply, which has been provided as much by economic determination as by nature.

We need look back no further than 50 years to find beef cattle unrecognizable from the hybridized breeds available to the abattoir of today. Prior to 1930, our major cattle production was range-fed on Johnson and Sudan grass, both high in nitriloside content, which remained residually in the meat production. The animals stood six feet at the shoulder and took up to four years to mature to slaughtering age. How different today is the feed-lot animal! Approximately four and one-half feet at the shoulder with a square and boxy configuration, it is slaughtered at the age of 18 to 24 months, following a chemically-controlled feeding program containing antibiotics and chemicals to force every ounce of weight increase at the least cost.

It is estimated that 75 percent of all beef sold in America today has been fed dietylstilbestrol, a synthetic hormonal fattening agent known to be possibly carcinogenic. The flagrant misuse of drugs in livestock production is flirting with tragedy that could make thalidomide seem insignificant. Some feed-lots actually feed ground newsprint, textile waste, and, in some cases, even polyethylene in an effort to reach market weight as quickly as possible. These artificially-fed animals have little opportunity to build protein muscle tissue. Soft, fat marbleized, meat is the palate standard of today.

In selecting meat for your table, if at all possible obtain naturally-raised, range-fed beef. This is still obtainable in many butcher shops if you specifically order it in advance. Many suburban communities are like mini-farms with inhabitants who raise three or four head of cattle for self use and are willing to sell quarters or sides for your freezer storage. A request at the local cold storage plant will provide you with a source for naturally-raised beef. At first, this meat will seem tough compared to the marbleized products you may be used to, but the naturally excellent flavor more than makes up for this difference, and the necessary increased mastication allows the meat to be thoroughly mixed with the primary digestive juices, ensuring a more efficient, comfortable digestive process.

The naturally-raised beef you obtain will have residual nitrilosides in the meat to a degree more or less depending upon the feed, but always more than feed-lot-produced animals that completely lack this cancer protective factor.

We are often asked specifically about organ meats. At one time in our biological history, these were unquestionably the most nourishing portion of the animal. Native cultures that do not domesticate, but rather hunt for their meat animals, still consider the liver, kidneys and other vital organs the supreme delicacy.

Unfortunately, these are the organs that attempt to screen the animals against many of the toxic substances forced upon them. As a consequence, most commercially-available organ meats contain the potentially carinogenic substances we are trying to avoid. When purchasing organ meats, bear in mind they should be from extremely young animals, calves and kids, where slaughter has occurred before toxic buildup has commenced.

Although man is omnivorous and meat may be included in his diet, if desired, this must be understood within the context of man's inherited biological experience. Primitive man's principal source of meat protein was the few small birds, reptiles and fish that he was physically able to capture. These small animals are composed of protein whose structure is far more easily accepted and digested by our systems. Perhaps the most easily digested and least toxic is fish. In spite of occasional unwarranted scare stories in our newspapers about high mercury or lead poisoning, fish are still the food source that civilization has been least able to contaminate. Ocean fish continue to exist in an environment subject to the natural food chain. Man has succeeded in making inedible some previously available lake, river and off-shore scavenger fish, but, generally speaking, fish is an easily digested source of protein that does not rob the body of its essential enzyme protection.

Chicken and other fowl are also easily digested. However, the economic requirement of rapid growth to slaughter weight subjects these animals to the same diets of medicated feed as cattle. Whenever possible, try to obtain barnyard-raised fowl from the same sources as mentioned for beef.

Meat should be used primarily as a condiment to flavor casseroles and vegetable dishes, rather than as a main course or focal point for each meal.

Our rule of thumb — to eat as close to the metabolic experiences of ancient man as possible — dictates to us that the animal protein contained in a Bio-X Diet should consist principally of fish and chicken, but even these in limited quantity. On rare occasion, our ancestors did obtain a satiating supply of red meat. During these infrequent instances the meat was most likely eaten to the exclusion of all other foods.

There is no metabolic reason why you cannot, from time to time, enjoy an occasional steak or piece of roast beef. Consider this "recreation eating." Try to restrict these occasions to no more than two or three times a month, and then limit your intake of other food categories. Since meat is the most slowly digested, if it is followed by quantities of fruit and vegetables they may remain above the meat and putrefy before digestion is completed.

The same general rule applied to lamb and game meats as to beef. Pork should be kept at an absolute minimum because of its extremely high fat content and difficult digestibility.

The Bio-X Diet does not call for fanaticism — just the continual referral to the common sense of our historical biologic experience.

We suggest the total protein intake be reduced to under 15 percent of the total nutritional intake, the majority of this coming from vegetable sources. The high-protein myth that only meat makes muscle tissue and the majority of body substance is protein (therefore, animal protein intake must be maintained at a high level to replenish these cells) is a totally fallacious theory foisted upon a gullible public by the meat industry. It is biologically incompatible with our digestive capabilities, which can obtain the same body-building nutrient from complex carbohydrates. Moreover, it places unanticipated stresses on the system that result, unquestionably, in many of our degenerative diseases, including, principally, cancer.

Inasmuch as the USDA includes eggs in its meat group, words are in order about this once-considered perfect, and complete, food that in recent years has become so maligned as to be recommended for elimination from the diet by both orthodox and preventive medicine.

Both sides of the war between the egg industry and the American Heart Association have produced series upon series of laboratory and clinical data that appear long on prejudice and short on science. We hesitate to quote either side, since equal and opposite data can be obtained from both. Certain facts do emerge:

The egg is high in cholesterol, averaging 275 mg. the average American diet has been determined to contain approximately 800 mg. per day. Obviously, eggs are a major contributor. Elimination of eggs, organ meat and whole milk and butter will reduce the intake to as low as 100 to 150 mg. per day. This is substantially less than the 1 to 2 grams the body manufactures each day. In addition to cholesterol, the egg contains zinc, iron, sulphur, and many trace elements which build native cholesterol into steroid hormones and other forms of body resistances to disease. It is interesting that lecithin contained in egg yolk has actually been demonstrated to dissolve serum cholesterol.

Certainly, unplanned excesses of any substance in the blood serum may lead to serious consequences. However, we must not overlook the necessity of maintaining normal amounts of these same substances. Cholesterol in proper proportions has a biological import that is only recently coming to light.

Substantial evidence, now being accumulated, suggests the possibility that the nervous drive and energy of some super achievers in our society are the result of their ability to maintain high cholesterol.

Of most interest to our cancer prevention research is the statistical result of a series of tests conducted under the auspices of the American Heart Association (AHA) on 500 males with abnormally high serum cholesterol levels. These subjects were placed on a cholesterol-lowering diet and observed against a non-diet control group for a period of five years. The results, as published, were as the AHA had predicted, an appreciable lessening of heart attacks within the diet group. There the matter rested until the spring of 1980 when a more in-depth investigation of the health of the subjects was computerized.

To the chagrin of the researchers, while the incidence of heart disease appeared lower among the subjects who were placed on a cholesterol-lowering diet, and observed against the non-diet control group, the incidence of cancer among the dieting group was almost four times that of the group that did not attempt reduction in serum levels.

This suggests once again that it is not what you eat that causes cancer, but what you do not eat that reduces your natural resistance to the disease. The research on these test groups is still continuing.

Many of the nutrients within the egg (niacin, magnesium, natural carbohydrates) are negatively associated with cancer as well as arteriosclerosis. Eggs, by themselves, are not the culprits in excessive levels of cholesterol. Only when the diet consists mainly of foods not having the trace elements and lacking in unrefined complex carbohydrates and the cholesterol-balancing dietary fiber do excessively high levels occur.

A common-sense solution to this nutritional controversy may be determined by referring to man's original blueprint and operating instructions as provided by our Creator.

Eggs were available to our aboriginal ancestors on a seasonal basis, but only infrequently due to the inaccessibility of most nesting areas.

Modern man has domesticated fowl. This increased the availability of eggs many-fold. The highly mechanized and advertised egg industry of the U.S. has upped the consumption even more. We believe blame for heart disease has been unduly placed on the egg to the detriment of its protective attributes in nutrition. It would be wise to concentrate on correcting an otherwise poor diet and retain a moderate quantity of this almost complete nutritional food source.

In the crisis diet period, the elimination of eggs and their animal protein content is essential. For normal cancer prevention we recommend the inclusion of one or two eggs per day or seven per week. At 275 mg. of cholesterol each, this is not an excessive amount if the remainder of the diet is well balanced.

Milk:

The arguments for the nutritional benefits of milk continue to wax and wane, centered mainly on lactose intolerance exhibited by many persons, the high cholesterol content, and milk's mucus-forming tendency. These are balanced against the nutritional content.

As to lactose sensitivity, many individuals with lactose intolerance will reject pasteurized milk naturally, or should consult their nutritionist.

Pasteurized milk is good for corporate profits, bad for consumer health. Pasteurized milk can sit on your grocer's shelf without spoiling because it has had the life force removed from it. The heating of milk during pasteurization destroys much of its natural content of vitamin C, vitamin B-1, vitamin B-12, calcium, phosphorus and iodine, it destroys 90% of the enzymes that help the human body utilize proteins, fats, sugars, starch, phosphorus and calcium. Furthermore regular pasteurized milk is tested for cleanliness only twice a month. Alta-Dena certified raw milk is tested daily.

We can find no reason to exclude certified raw milk, once the fat content is removed, from the cancer-preventive diet. Milk in its fresh, natural state has a better taste and contains the properties important to good nutrition that are altered when milk is pasteurized and homogenized. If milk appeals to your palate, skimmed and raw milk is an acceptable beverage. We definitely recommend certified raw milk, as opposed to the pasteurized, homogenized, fortified brands on the market, for its digestibility. It is, of course, important that the milk you obtain comes from a naturally-raised, disease-free herd. The brand available in most health food stores is Alta-Dena Dairy certified raw milk. We unhesitatingly recommend the quality of their products.

Vegetables, Fruits and Grains:

In the Bio-X Diet, we have combined the category of vegetables and fruits with the grain category. These two divisions were, as should be expected, originated by the USDA on an agricultural rather than a nutritional basis. The bulk of our nutrition should be from foods within this all-inclusive group — all the carbohydrates, protein and fats required for complete nutrition. The similarity of its content and necessity in the diet preclude any need for separation.

Before considering vegetables, fruits and grains as they apply to the prevention of cancer, a most important word should be said about their preparation.

Preparation:

When ancient man first was using the body mechanism we later inherited, fire was a fearful thing. Neither the knowledge nor the utensils were available then that have given modern man the ability to burn, boil, and scorch. Edible plants and grains were eaten very close to their natural state; seldom were they so plentiful as to be dissected into parts. Our Creator in His infinite wisdom, designed perfect foods, the sum of whose parts appears to perfectly match our digestive abilities and nutritional needs. The fact that modern man destroys much of his food by heat, coats it with digestion-preventive oil, and mechanically extracts or chemically adds to much of the rest is a tragedy of civilization. Food processing tends to transform protective foods into threats to the body's defense mechanism. Cooking often renders the most protective food indigestible and enzyme impotent. The advantages of cooking food in a civilized society must not be totally overlooked, however, and in some cases cooked food is dictated by modern civilized lifestyles.

The consumption of large quantities of raw food requires a vigorous digestion. Primitive man's prodigious physical activities to sustain a constant search for food and avoidance of danger promoted good metabolism. Civilized man, who uses his mind rather than his body, suffers with an accordingly less vigorous digestion and longer bowel transit period.

Heating food can accomplish several requirements of modern civilization. When plant foods are cooked, heat causes the starch within the cell to swell. This opens the fibrous cell wall, releasing the nutrients within and making them more readily available to the digestive process. This is particularly important in the case of many of our hard cereal grains, legumes and lentils.

In terms of quantity, more food can be ingested when its bulk is reduced by heat. With many modern vegetables deficient in vitamins and minerals, cooking effectively increases our ability to obtain adequate nutritional value. Additionally, the breaking down of the plant cell makes up for our lack of complete mastication, so important to primitive man; he, no doubt, ate in a manner far different from the hustle-and-bustle, bolt-eating habits of most modern-day Americans. In the case of meats, heat converts the connective tissue to a soft consistency that would otherwise be extremely difficult to chew and would make abnormally difficult digestive demands on our body.

The appropriate degree of cooking should depend on plant toughness or the amount of fiber, its digestibility and, of course, the constitution and way of life of the individual. As much as possible when cooking, use only low heat to reduce bulk of food intake without destroying the enzyme and vitamin content. As a general rule, if the color of the vegetable remains true, the vitamin and enzyme content will remain at near normal potency. When the vegetable changes color, or even hue, valuable nutrition has been lost. Steaming or light wok cooking (Chinese style) does the least nutritional damage; frying and broiling the most.

Anti-Cancer Nutrient in Seeds, Nuts, Beans:

Many fine books on plant nutrient content are available at any health food store. And, of course, this information is available through your nutritionally-oriented medical professional. Of major interest to this volume are the grains and plants that formerly provided our extrinsic cancer protection but have been eliminated from man's food chain.

We have already mentioned the nitriloside grasses no longer generally available to range-fed cattle, and the loss of this residual source in our meat supply.

The richest source of nitrilosides or amygdalin occurs in the seeds and kernels of all of our common fruits, with the exception of the citrus family. Even in the case of citrus, amygdalin is found in the seeds of the original African varieties — another example of how hybridization has increased size, sugar content, and yield, but manipulated nutritional content to our detriment.

In less sophisticated and privileged societies than our own, where each morsel of food must be utilized, the seeds of the fruit are the most highly prized portion. Where plenty exists, modern man throws away the core or kernel and with it one of the most nutritionally important foods — amygdalin.

Watch any ape, monkey or chimpanzee in the zoo. These closest biological cousins of man, when offered fruit, will instinctively tear open the sweet fleshy portion and crack open the kernel. Nature compels them to eat whole foods in spite of the fact they may never have been given that type of food before.

Certainly our biological experience calls for us to follow the example of animals and our own ancestors. Get into the habit of eating the whole fruit and eat it often.

When you eat an apple, do not throw the core away. Eat it right along with the rest of the fruit. Do exactly the same with grapes, and melons. You are going to discover that the seeds add a pleasant, crunchy texture to the fruit. And the very slight bitterness of their amygdalin content is totally masked by the sweetness of the flesh. The masticated seeds are an excellent additional fiber supply.

For those fruits having kernels protected by a hard outer shell, such as cherry, peach and apricot, man does not possess the jaw structure to open them as animals can. One of the few nutritional advantages of civilization is the development of more sophisticated methods of opening a seed than banging it between two rocks. For modern man we suggest a hammer or nutcracker. Many individuals will not take the time, and for them civilization also provides another answer — the health food store where, if it has not been subjected to FDA harrassment, apricot kernels will be available in bulk or 1-lb. bags.

Of all the seed kernels and plants, the apricot kernel — containing approximately three percent by weight of amygdalin — is our richest readily available source of amygdalin. The apricot has long been a staple in the diet of many Mediterranean and Himalayan peoples. Where they are eaten, the incidence of cancer is relatively unknown. In spite of the always-unfounded rumors circulated (and inspired from time to time, we believe) by the resistors of natural medicine, apricot kernels are not only non-toxic when eaten in normal amounts, but, when prepared and eaten properly, can be delicious. To many persons it is a taste that must be acquired. Personally, I find that apricot kernels, when prepared as a trail mix with raisins, a few chopped dates and a little coconut, are delicious. Several kernel recipes are included in our second section.

We are often asked by individuals who wish to maintain an aggressive prevention program how many kernels they should take each day. A standard answer would be to eat as many of the kernels as would normally be eaten of the fruit. If a more exacting rule of thumb is desired, eat one kernel for every 10 pounds of body weight.

If you do nothing else that we recommend in this chapter, get some kernels and return this rich source of nitriloside to your diet. For cancer prevention it is natural — and far less expensive than reinforcing your preventive diet with extracted amygdalin in tablet form.

Virtually all seeds and nuts, with the exception of the peanut (actually not a true nut), contain varying amounts of amygdalin and should be included, in liberal amounts, in your diet. We refer, of course, to raw nuts — not the deep-fried, roasted and salted varieties. Heat will reduce the effective amygdalin content and destroy the enzymes.

The oil content of raw nuts will in time become rancid if shelled and exposed to the air. We suggest that all raw nuts, including apricot kernels, be refrigerated or kept in the freezer.

It is sometimes overlooked that beans and grains are actually seeds. Like nuts, they are the embryonic plant reproduction entity containing all the elements for a new plant. They are our richest sources of all nutrition including cancer-protective nitrilosides.

All whole, unrefined grains, with one major exception, wheat, are rich sources of nitrilosides.

Unfortunately, only the primitive forms of wheat contain amygdalin. Like the citrus plant, hybridization has increased yield at the expense of some of wheat's otherwise extremely nutritional attributes.

Among all grains, the one highest in amygdalin content is millet, a delicious cereal grain which was a staple of the American diet in the 1800s. With the advent of refined white flour, it has gradually disappeared from our tables.

Unfortunatey, millet's departure has been accompanied by that of other whole grains that used to serve as breakfast and baking staples but have now been replaced by refined and packaged cereals that have less food value than the boxes they come in, and by store-bought baked products that, even when fortified, fail to provide adequate nutrition.

Equal with unrefined grains as sources of nitrilosides — and equally depleted from our modern diet — are the lentils and legumes.

Beans, not only because they are high in protein content but because of their capability of lengthy bulk storage without deterioration, were a staple food until the early 1900s. As commercial canning, refrigeration, and rapid transportation made more fragile vegetables available on a year-around basis, beans became regarded as poor man's food. Our newly-affluent society of the 1900s rejected such low-priced plebian fare, and with their rejection went yet another source of nitrilosides.

The trend to prepackaging, convenience foods, and the reduction of fiber content, was a hallmark of our emerging opulence in the early 1900s. It was, indeed, a diet revolution and its ultimate effect has been a frightful increase in cancer fatalities.

CHAPTER 11:

The Nutrition Revolution of the 1900s

"No wealth accumulated in our lifetime can compensate us for the premature failure of our bodies"

Floyd Weston
Nevada Clinic of
Preventive Medicine

In spite of the American Cancer Society's continual insistence that it is the carcinogens of modern society which are responsible for the 1-in-4 cancer rate, statistics indicate otherwise. Studies by the NCI go back only to 1937, but data from the following years to 1969 indicate only a six percent cancer increase during that period. Orthodoxy agrees that most cancer requires at least 15 years before the overt exhibition of symptoms. It must be concluded, therefore, that the high incidence of the disease among U.S. whites in 1937 was precipitated by factors in existence in 1922. If statements propagated by the NCI and ACS about the carinogenic causes of cancer are true, the causes could not have been food additives, farm chemicals, radiation, environmental pollution and high levels of stress, all of which collectively bear the chief brunt of those two agencies' accusations. Like cancer, these factors are linked to a high living standard but, unlike cancer, they were insignificant in 1920. Logical consideration of these facts renders establishment medicine's position on the causes of cancer totally untenable.

What was occurring in the white civilized society of the 1920s was a nutritional revolution, one that was eliminating from our diet the nitrilosides contained in lentils, legumes and simple grains, extracting the fiber from our other grains and vegetables, changing our meat production and, all the while, increasing our intake of sugar and reducing fiber intake with the newly developed processes of squeezing sugar from beets and oil from vegetables.

There is further statistical indication that the real cause of America's cancer epidemic is the reduction in our natural defenses brought about by the aforementioned diet revolution, rather than by environmental carcinogens. Ample evidence may be derived by using our population of black citizens as a control group for historical analysis.

During the early 1900s, the black population, centered mainly in the South, continued their diet of millet, blackeyed peas, sorghum, beans, molasses — all poor-folk food, but nitriloside-rich nutrition. In 1937, the rate of cancer among black males was two-thirds less than among their white counterparts. But since World War II, dietary habits of blacks have changed radically, the result of a tremendous increase in economic opportunity for the black population. Affluence consigned soul food to nostalgia and with its loss has come increasing incidence of malignancy. Today both black and white populations are subject to the same fearful 1-in-4 statistics.

These statistical facts emphasize the nutritional logic that we will maintain our body's defenses against cancer not be eliminating carcinogens, but by returning to our biological experience and restoring to our diet the high-nitrilosides, fiber grains and legumes of earlier time.

How to Increase Nitriloside Content

Happily, there is a method of substantially increasing the nitriloside content of grains and legumes even more. As stated previously, seeds, nuts and beans are the embryonic, all inclusive pattern of the subsequent plant. During the very early stages of germination, when cell proliferation is at its greatest, the young plant may double in weight during a 24-hour period. The quantity of nitrilosides, vitamins and minerals increases with the same proliferation — doubling, tripling, and even quadrupling the original seed content. The sprouts of alfalfa, mung beans, rye and bamboo are all vitamin- enzyme- and nitriloside-rich. By all means, purchase a book on sprouting at your health food store. The methods are simple, and the results are a delicious and inexpensive sources of cancer preventive amygdalin and enzymes.

In addition to our richest amygdalin sources — sprouts, grains, seeds, nuts and legumes — nitrilosides are contained in over 1,100 varietal plants. A list of many of these foods is contained in the Appendix. We must, however, consider another problem of our generation — availability of proper whole foods.

Naturally-Cultivated Produce Is Best

For most of us it is no longer possible to either raise or forage for our food supply. Our hunting ground is the local supermarket, and hunting isn't so good this season. Eliminate the prepared, the packaged, the sugared, the preserved, and very little is left. The produce department, while its contents may still look crisp, colorful and delicious, contains a preponderance of vegetables raised under what can only be regarded as artificial environments. Unnatural fertilizers and growth stimulants have, at best, robbed many plants of their natural nutrients. At worst, pesticides have actually introduced poisons with unquestionably deleterious effects on body mechanism.

Many of the most nutritious and necessary plants and sources for individual nutrients are no longer readily available. This problem may be eliminated by finding a store where organic natural produce is for sale. Sometimes this can be accomplished by demanding that your present green-grocer inform you as to where his produce is obtained and how it is raised. He will shortly cooperate with his knowledgeable customer because these products are available in the wholesale market for the retailer who demands them. Demand always creates supply.

What faith we might retain in the good intentions for the health of each citizen exhibited by our U.S. Department of Health and Department of Agriculture is totally destroyed when we consider their final two recommendations for inclusion in the USDA Fitness Diet: sugar and fat.

Sugar

Less than 300 years ago, refined sugar was produced in extremely small quantity and considered an addictive medicinal. All of man's sweetening needs were provided in the fruit nectars, seasonably obtained, and the honey he had learned to produce domestically in small amounts. Perhaps the most physically-devastating addition to the hazards of modern living is the availability and dietary inclusion of excessive amounts of sugar.

The USDA includes five ounces of sugar (almost one-third of a pound) per day in its Fitness Diet. Hardly a surprise when they have also recommended refined grains in their regimen. The political and economic pressure to promote the products of our giant sugar refining industry are no less than the political homage due to the millers or our grain, the producers of breakfast cereals, and the commercial baking companies.

What can we say about sugar that has not been said? Through its role in hypoglycemia, sugar is responsible for a host of neurotic behavioral symptoms. Even orthodoxy has linked sugar with diseases ranging from diabetes to cataracts. There is little we can add to what has already been written. Sugar serves no known dietary need and it is more addictive than many prescriptive drugs. The increased consumption of sugar in the United States since World War I has been proportional to increases in degenerative diseases.

The body's protective mechanism can handle limited amounts of refined sugar but, by all means, it should be kept at a minimum. In almost every instance, cancer is accompanied by an additional metabolic disease that has placed stress on the body. In many instances, excess sugar was one of the root causes of the disease that was a precursor of cancer. In addition, sugar has the ability to alter the nature and amount of intestinal bacteria, impairing both digestion and the synthesis of essential cancer-resisting nitrilosides.

Our metabolic defenses can protect us to an extent beyond the anticipated stress of our biological experience. But our systems were not designed for excessive cupcakes, Twinkies and candy bars. The Bio-X Diet, therefore, excludes such unnatural products except as very occasional treats.

Fats

Fat is a necessary part of human nutrition. However, primitive societies (with a few exceptions, e.g., Eskimos, as previously noted) include substantially less in their diets than consumed by modern man; and fat, when consumed, was part of the naturally-balanced diet of availability. The nutritional need of humans for fat, as determined by man's biological experience, is included in the Bio-X Diet. It is fully satisfied by the recommended content of grains, vegetables and lean meat. In these natural sources, fat is combined in balanced amounts with protein carbohydrates and fiber.

One of man's earliest adventures in devastating his natural nutrition was the discovery of methods to separate pure oil from its vegetable or animal source by squeezing, churning, or heating. Modern mechanization has refined these techniques further with powerful presses that turn corn, peanuts, and even wheat into refined table oils, eliminating the natural balance of fiber bulk and other nutrients.

No less authoritative clinicians than M. W. Sterns, Jr., M.D., Chief of Colon-Rectal Service at Memorial Sloan-Kettering, and E. L. Winder, M.D., president of the American Health Foundation, (and even American Cancer Society bulletins) have in recent years warned of the danger of our unnaturally-high fat diets as a cause of cancer.

Nutritionally-oriented physicians have been aware of this direct connection for many years. And they have warned against the USDA's continued inclusion of fats as 49 percent of the total caloric intake of their recommended diet.

The brilliant pioneer, Dr. Max Gerson, while being maligned by the orthodoxy of his time, cited evidence of clinical recurrence of regressed tumors when patients were fed fats. These continuing clinical observations have had prior support in irrefutable laboratory research. Rats fed a commercial dye all developed liver tumors when fed on a diet containing 20 percent corn oil. High fat levels have raised the incidence of carcinogenic and spontaneous breast tumors in mice.

It is evident that fat not only lowers body resistance but is the carrier of fat-related carcinogens.

In spite of voluminous evidence that dietary fat causes more new cases of cancer each year than smoking, the USDA continues to suggest that fat should constitute almost half of one's recommended caloric intake! The same political machinery that dictates continued subsidization of the tobacco industry prevents the USDA from eliminating fats or at least educating our population to this tremendous dietary hazard. It would be commendable, indeed, for the American Cancer Society to supplement their effective anti-smoking campaign with one against the equally dangerous ingestion of fat.

High fat has been implicated in coronary heart disease, multiple sclerosis, gallstones, arthritis and strokes, in addition to cancer.

We take a major step in reduction of fat from the Euro-American diet when we limit our intake of animal protein. The elimination of whole milk further reduces fat intake toward acceptable levels.

Where possible, we recommend the elimination of refined oils such as peanut butter, olive oil and corn oil; polyunsaturated or not, it makes no difference. In fact, in spite of the recent publicity concerning the polyunsaturated oils, they do not exist abundantly in nature; and if, indeed, they are not harmful, they will be the only exception we know of to the axiomatic fact that whatever food man manipulates becomes nutritionally undesirable. Sooner or later we expect science to discover some error in its dietary recommendations and return us to natural oils.

We do not feel that total elimination of oil is necessary. But certainly, deep-fried foods should be eliminated, along with heavily-oil-polluted salad dressings. Butter's plastic counterpart, margarine, should be substantially reduced. Limited use of butter in stir cooking, baking and other food preparation is acceptable. The reason we need not entirely eliminate refined fat, besides acknowledging it as a palatable addition to many foods, is that the major dietary danger posed by the unbalanced nutritional intake of an extracted fat can be eliminated when we return, by way of the Bio-X Diet, that element of whole foods which has been eliminated by the oil- and fat-extracting processes.

This postulate introduces one of the most important components, along with the nitrilosides and enzymes of the Bio-X Diet, as applied to cancer prevention.

Fiber

Traditionally, all the elements of a diet necessary for complete nutrition are contained in three categories: Protein, Carbohydrate and Fat. Within these divisions are all the enzymes, all the calories, all of the vitamins necessary, with the addition of water, to sustain a well-balanced diet. Modern civilization ignores, and in many instances eliminates, a fourth important food factor from our total nutrition. That missing ingredient is fiber, without which no diet can be truly balanced. Failure to include this important factor results in an improperly functioning digestive system. The inevitable result is degenerative disease. Often that disease will be cancer.

Consistently, where researchers have found high cancer death rates in populations with a singularly high intake in one type of food, be it meat or refined carbohydrates or cholesterol, those populations have excluded appreciable amounts of fiber from their diets.

We have spoken of the dietary revolution that occurred in the early 1900s. It is estimated that the dietary fiber intake of the average individual living in Europe or the United States is only one-fifth what it was 100 years ago. The primary cause has been a drop in bulk consumption of seed grains from 350 pounds per year to less than 150 — much of this refined — and the inclusion in the diet of bulk meats and refined sugar products which bring calories but no fiber.

Again, a perfect analogy for the dietary role of fiber may be found in petroleum engineering — the improvements in engine design, fuel and lubricants by which our automobiles have been made to operate more efficiently.

Basically refined oil and gasoline will temporarily provide satisfactory engine operation. But without the inclusion of various detergents and blends of catalytic additives ranging from graphite to lead, the cylinder walls will scuff, the valves become clogged with sludge, and the spark plugs will foul, all resulting in an inefficiently-functioning mechanism that will eventually break down.

So, too, non-nutritive fiber was included in man's natural fuel supply as an aid in the digestive function toward perfect metabolism of our food. Removing fiber results in the malfunction our digestive processes, leading to a degenerative disease which may well be cancer.

For most of man's biological experience, fiber in the diet was not in question. Each morsel of natural food contained fiber. All foods were eaten whole, including their seeds and hulls. Our modern proclivity for taste, texture and appearance has neglected metabolic needs by the substitution of bulk foods which contain little fiber.

The primary function of fiber is to facilitate elimination of waste products from the body. When little fiber is in the diet, residue reaching the colon does not move easily. In modern societies, some individuals require as long as ten days for a small amount of residue to pass out in the stool. One week is not at all unusual, and 72 hours is considered, by orthodox medicine, to be more or less normal.

In Hunza or Abkasia, where all foods are unrefined, transit time of food through the intestinal tract may be as short as six hours. It is obvious that lack of fiber, which can treble or quadruple bowel transit time, gives the toxins and carcinogens present in our modern foods three and four times as long to be absorbed in the body.

In and of itself, unnaturally extended transit in the bowels allows the best of foods to putrefy and produce toxemic substances that are carcinogenic.

Laboratory studies at Knarfy Bnettirw, Indonesia, have shown that a diet high in refined carbohydrates induced cancer in mice. With this same diet, but including a substantial portion of crude fiber, the incidence of cancer was substantially reduced. These laboratory studies of dietary fiber substantiate the theory that fat and refined carbohydrates can be included in limited amounts if we replace in our diet the fiber these foods have excluded by reason of their own bulk and lack of inherent contents.

Unprocessed crude plant fiber, particularly in the case of fat intake, keeps down serum cholesterol. How this is metabolically accomplished is still unclear. It appears the liver breaks down cholesterol to produce bile which is secreted into the intestines. There is substantial evidence that fiber in the bowel increases demand for bile, which leads to its increased production and, hence, removal of cholesterol from the blood by the liver.

Field studies by Dr. Nil Knarf of the rural African tribesmen who exist on a high milk and meat diet, show extremely low serum cholesterol and diverticular disease. Their diet includes about 25 grams per day of fiber, at least five times that of Western civilization. These same natives, like all populations subsisting on a traditional diet of whole foods, are free of colon cancer, a disease that plagues Western man. It has been found that bile can be altered by certain bacteria to produce carcinogenic substances. These bacteria are far less common in the intestines of high-fiber-eating people.

In addition to the indirect carcinogenic result of low fiber and lengthened bowel transit, bacterial flora — necessary to the metabolic breakdown of amygadalin for the performance of its protective function — maintain higher concentrations if there is normal fiber intake in the intestinal environment.

Orthodoxy's speculation on all of the above has led in recent years to a flurry of high-fiber diets. These diets all specify the consumption of unnatural refined grains and high meat intake, with the simple addition of huge amounts of wheat bran. This, in itself, may produce unnatural results which, once again, underscores the need for having a perfect balance of nutrition planned into our natural food supply.

Bran contains phytic acid. When more is included in the diet than is naturally contained in the whole grains, fruits and leaves, it can chelate or bind materials during the digestive process that removes them from the body, thus producing deficiencies in such vital minerals as zinc and calcium.

Additional laboratory experiments indicate that while artificially adding bran to an otherwise depleted diet has some good effects, it cannot match those of whole fiber-rich foods. Rice bran, added to a starch diet, reduced blood cholesterol in test animals from 348 to 255. When whole grain was used, the level dropped to 165. Obviously, there are also other indigestible plant substances besides bran that are of equal importance in dropping cholesterol levels, and these are eliminated when the natural food is refined.

The Bio-X Diet returns natural fiber to our nutritional process, first by reducing the bulk of meat intake, and secondly, by replacing this bulk with beans, seeds and unrefined grains in a proportion natural to one's biologic experience. This is a most important preventive to the digestive malfunctions that are a leading source of carcinogens and their cancerous results.

Water

Important as it is to abide by biological experience in the selection of our food, equal consideration should be given to the daily intake of life-sustaining water. Sounds simple enough. But is it? Unfortunately, water — like the air we breathe — has become contaminated by metropolitan pollutants and chemicals. Not to just an objectionable degree, but to a point where this natural resource, so essential to life, may also become the instrument of its destruction.

Modern society has outgrown its dependence on natural sources of water — crystal-clear springs and cool, deep lakes maintained in pristine, unspoiled freshness by nature. Not only has our water become polluted by the wastes of industry, but in recent years the residual insecticides and fertilizers of agriculture have been appearing in increasing amounts in even our deep water supplies. Many of the substances that seep into municipal water resources cannot be filtered away. Chlorine and a host of other chemicals are added to prevent contaminants from causing viral disease. The long-range effect of many of these additives can be likened to a metabolic time bomb, its inexorable ticking becoming more and more audible to those who realize what these chemicals can do to the body.

In recent years the addition of fluoride has spawned government-enforced medication on whole populations where freedom of choice is denied. There can no longer be doubt that fluoride is carcinogenic when taken over an extended period.[1] Not only is the water we are provided municipally harmful because of additives and original pollutants, but the delivery system of lead, copper and aluminum piping is, in and of itself, a provider of the heavy metals that can be absolutely deadly when cellularly absorbed.

Investment in a water distiller, or the purchase of bottled water, is the only way to avoid this continuous assault on our immune system. We cannot overemphasize the importance of pure water. It cleanses the body and prevents toxic buildup. The traditional admonition to drink at least eight glasses of pure water a day remains excellent advice. Certain commercial spring waters on the market contain mineral contents that may be particularly beneficial. Your nutrition professional will be able to advise on local availability.

A final brief word on the toxins that may be absorbed into food during preparation. It would be a shame to have purchased organically-grown produce which was then combined and prepared with pure water and then complete the preparation in utensils of copper, aluminum, tin, or Teflon that could, themselves, provide the heavy metals and contaminants so devastating to a healthy, natural metabolism. Stainless steel, glass, or ceramic cookware are the concluding link from farm to tongue that provides the contaminant-free sustenance required to maintain the cancer-resisting immune system you inherited from biological experience.

Conclusions

The Bio-X Diet as applied to the prevention of cancer is supported equally by simple logic, animal research and empirical evaluation of cultures which maintain a close adherence to these dietary principles and remain cancer free.

To apply the Bio-X Diet in our everyday lives, we need only refer to a simple rule: eat as close to the biological habits of our prehistoric antecedents as is possible in a modern world. It is this biologic experience that our bodies are designed to utilize in selecting and preparing our natural food supply.

We know of no type of food or food preparation that, if nutritionally questioned, can be subjected to this test and provide a resultant answer that would not be correct for proper metabolism. If you are ever in doubt about a particular food substance or its method of preparation, simply ask yourself if it is a whole food and if aboriginal society could or would have included it in a diet of the time. If the answer is "no," then 99 times out of 100 that particular food would be harmful if consumed on a continuing basis.

As an example, consider the beverage coffee. Would or could aboriginal man have roasted the bean? Would he have then ground it, leached it with hot water and finally thrown away the spent residue? Of course not. This simple mental exercise has shown you that coffee is a totally unnatural food unknown to our body's biological experience and most likely will be harmful if consumed regularly. As a matter of fact, coffee may be responsible for a host of metabolic disorders, from hypertension to heart disease. Recent clinical studies suggest a very evident carcinogenic effect with a particularly strong linkage to cancer of the pancreas.

Fortunately, because we must live in this mechanized, urbanized society, our bodies have the built-in tolerance and protective systems to adjust to unanticipated dietary variances, as well as recreational exceptions, that are part and parcel of a modern world. This is particularly true when we return to our diet the nitriloside-containing foods that are extrinsic defenses necessary to protect us from cancer.

The Bio-X Diet is, therefore, a diet of common sense, not of asceticism, total self denial, charts and scales. By returning such important food factors as amygdalin (nitriloside) and fiber, a protective balance is maintained that allows temperate ingestion of many foods that would otherwise be carcinogenic.

In essence, the Bio-X Diet for cancer prevention provides the following contrasts with the average American diet, as suggested and recommended by the USDA in their Fitness Diet:

1. Reduce meat consumption to approximately one-fourth of total protein intake. The Bio-X Diet contains no more than ½ lb. per day, including one egg. Animal protein should be primarily fowl and fish, which makes the least demand on the digestive processes. Red meat should be eaten only occasionally, and then it should be as lean as possible, preferably ranch-fed. Unlike the USDA Fitness Diet, we do not recommend a minimum daily meat consumption. Quite the contrary. Practically all protein requirements can be obtained from our grains and vegetables; and it is advisable to maintain meat consumption as low as possible. Just by cutting consumption of red meat in-half, and substituting fowel or fish we cut carcinogenic fat 30 percent and free the pancreatic enzymes for their role in the cancer suppression metabolism.

2. All dairy products should be low-fat or fat-free and preferably unpasteurized. This reduces daily fat intake an additional 12 percent from the USDA diet. The advisability of excluding milk where other degenerative diseases may exist should be discussed with your holistic physician or nutritionist. Many times the problems found with pasteurized products will be non-existent with raw certified dairy products.

3. Vegetables and fruit consumption must be increased to become, whenever possible, the center focus of the meal, rather than the side dish. Heavy emphasis is placed upon returning the high nitriloside legumes to everyday inclusion in the diet as a meat substitute. Seeds will no longer be thrown away, but considered part of the whole fruit or vegetable. Vegetables will be cooked as little as possible, not deep-oil-fried, or similarly detroyed and coated. The complex unrefined carbohydrates should become 75 percent of total nutritional intake and will capably supply all but a small portion of our need for protein.

4. Grains: The consumption of unrefined grains should be at least tripled from USDA recommendations to a minimum of two large portions of whole grains per day with a heavy emphasis on the nitriloside grains, such as millet. Not only are the whole grains a rich source of amygdalin, but dietary fiber will be naturally increased.

On the Bio-X Diet the ordinary ingestion of fiber will increase from approximately 2.5 grams per day on the USDA Fitness Diet to 15 grams per day with a corresponding decrease in bowel transit time, a reduction in blood serum cholesterol, and much reduced opportunity for the toxemic effects of food putrefaction and its attendant carcinogenic effects.

5. Sugar: Wherever possible, eliminate or cut down on sugar and substitute natural fruit nectars, raisins, fruit, small quantities of honey. Sorghum syrup contains nitrilosides and should be the sweetner of first choice.

6. Fats: The additional fat category, as recommended by the USDA must be substantially reduced. However, the tremendous reduction achieved by substituting grains and legumes for meat, and the elimination of whole-milk products, has already reduced fat intake to near acceptable levels. While the Bio-X Diet does not recommend butter, olive oil, peanut oil, etc., the increased ingestion of dietary fiber enables the metabolism to anticipate the temperate use of oil in cooking, salad dressings, and as a light spread on whole-grain breads.

When the Bio-X Diet is compared directly with the recommended adult intake on the USDA diet, differences are immediately obvious. Total caloric intake is substantially lessened. Meat has been reduced from 61.2 percent of the protein source to less than one-fourth. This can, and should, if palatably possible, be reduced still further by increasing the consumption of vegetables and grains which, together on the Bio-X Diet, account for 63.4 percent of the protein intake.

Fat has been reduced from 31 percent to 10 percent of total nutrition and carbohydrates now account for 75 percent.

A most important difference between the two diets concerning cancer prevention cannot be determined by percentage of meat protein consumed but is of primary importance in providing our extrinsic protection against the disease. When meat is included in a meal, it will be primarily chicken, or fish. Infrequent portions of red meat will be as lean as possible. This reduces fat out of proportion with protein reduction. Pasteurized milk is good for corporate health, bad for consumer health. Pasteurization removes the life force and makes milk a dead product. Calves cannot live on pasteurized milk, they become mean and unmanagable. When dairy products are included by choice, they will now be fat free and certified raw.

Vegetables are to be eaten as near their natural whole state as possible; a high proportion of these will be plants and legumes containing large percentages of nitrilosides, which are neglected in the USDA diet plan.

Unlike the USDA diet, the basic Bio-X Diet accepts only whole, unrefined grains, seeds and nuts, with heavy emphasis on previously neglected grains high in nitrilosides. The increased fiber intake of whole grains speeds digestion, reduces cholesterol and permits proper metabolism of dietary fat. Sprouting will increase the vitamin, mineral and enzyme content of grains even far beyond their bulk increase, further reinforcing our natural immuno-suppression of cancer.

Obesity

Of vital importance in the prevention of malignancy is the statistically determined effect of obesity or overweight. Without exception, our prehistoric ancestors possessed lean and muscular bodies. Not only did their environment demand such a physique for survival, but their food supply was limited at times to the point of famine. In addition, it was naturally low in fat and completely lacking in cookies, soft drinks and ice cream.

We will not discuss here the benefits of fasting, as applied to modern man. There are many books explaining its benefits and, of course, a trained physician should be consulted before commencing such a program. The prevention of degenerative disease is, in large measure, dependent on maintaining our bodies in the lean condition of our biological experience. The Bio-X Diet will help its participant to maintain normal body weight by eliminating the dietary sources of much of modern man's weight problems.

We have referred in this book to the eating ceremony during which civilized man eats at specific times, regardless of his hunger or exercise-created need for additional caloric intake. Our culture has created food neurotics to whom gluttony is an emotional release, and food is a continually necessary palliative.

The Bio-X Diet is balanced nutritionally and can provide delicious and satisfying meals, examples of which will be given in the recipe section. The individual who continues, through habit, to ingest more calories than his or her body can utilize, even on this nutritionally sound diet, will still become obese.

Dr. Albert Tannenbaum has reported that many different types of mouse tumors and leukemia are inhibited by restricted food consumption. He has found no tumor that does not respond with lessening incidence of spontaneous occurrence when caloric intake is reduced. Dr. Jesse Greenstein confirmed these studies with his own research in which caloric restriction dropped breast cancers in one strain of mice from 38 percent to 0, and from 100 to 10 percent in another.

Dr. Tannenbaum also found the incidence of induced skin cancer in animals was substantially reduced, even when caloric restriction began long after the carcinogen had been applied.

While the reduction of food intake once a tumor commences does not lead to its disappearance, experience with animals shows that limiting food intake does appear to go a long way in preventing the disease. Life expectancy studies performed by major insurance companies confirm a corresponding correlation among overweight policy holders. The statistics are uncontestable. Cancer deaths per 100,000 population increase proportionately with excess weight.

Our biological experience was one of extensive physical activity with food consumed as necessary. To maintain a normal body weight, we must not only conform to the diet of biological experience, but must exercise as often as possible and allow the body to tell us what amounts of food it requires. Do not let habit, gluttony or social custom dictate an unnatural path to your physical deterioration.

Notes — CHAPTER ELEVEN

1. Dr. Dean Burk, Dr. J. Yamayanis. *Public Scrutiny,* June, 1979.

CHAPTER 12:

Supplementation

"The physician of tomorrow will be the nutritionist of today."

Thomas Edison

Medicine in the United States, for the most part, downplays the role of nutrition in the treatment of disease, or as a factor that causes it, and most often rejects the use of vitamin supplementation. Orthodoxy's line is that only the drugs produced by giant conglomerates are worthy of consideration. Interferon is the latest to be foisted on the nutritionally-uneducated physician and his patients by a multimillion-dollar publicity campaign that can only be viewed as the medical ripoff of the decade.

In defense of their lack of consideration of vitamins in a program of preventive health maintenance, orthodoxy points to magnificent hospitals and centers of medical research and education as proof that their science must be superior to any natural nutrition, or nutritional supplementation, in providing Americans with the finest health care in the world.

Unfortunately, their statements are not substantiated in fact. Males in the United States rank 18th in the world statistics of longevity. Females rank 10th, primarily because of our advances in obstetrical science, which have tremendously reduced death in childbirth.

Of the 17 nations whose male citizens outlive our own, all are culturally oriented to diets containing far higher amounts of unrefined complex carbohydrates and far less meat.

Our nation is advanced in the prevention of infant mortality, which makes our statistics on longevity from birth appear deceptively better than they actually are. We applaud the advances our physicians have made against childhood disease and in operating-room techniques that increase the expectancy of survival. The facts are, however, that once our citizens have reached maturity and have avoided traumatic disease or surgery, the rate of longevity shows no statistical increase over the last 50 years. Indeed, some medical statisticians actually detect a downturn.

We believe there is substantial evidence that a return to proper nutrition can reverse this trend. The physician of tomorrow will be educated in nutrition and the specific methods of supportive supplementation that will, as a consequence, be reflected in the increased health and longevity of our citizenry.

Even within the ranks of nutritionists, there are advocates of currently-voguish health food diets that reject the necessity of any dietary supplementation. These proponents maintain that all nutritional needs may be obtained from our natural food supply. In their eagerness to promote the total nutrition available in organically-grown produce and improved eating habits, they fail to consider that availability and obtainability are two vastly different things.

It has been previously pointed out that we are not what we eat, but rather what we can digest. The ability to metabolize and utilize what is available is the final determining factor in human nutrition. It varies greatly between individuals. In other words, even if nutritionally-adequate foods are available on our tables, all persons will not necessarily have the same ability to properly digest and metabolize them. Modern civilized man, in his urbanized, mechanized environment, has eliminated the laws of natural selection that governed the well-being of his ancient antecedents. No longer do only the physically strong and swift, who logically best convert food to energy, survive. In today's world, mental acumen may well prove even more contributory to longevity than physical ability.

We are all familiar with large families, military organizations, or similarly well-defined and structured populations and groups where available nutrition to all is identical, yet among their individual members there is a marked variance in disease resistances, stamina, energy levels, and many of the other standard measures of normal metabolism. Individuals who have inherently poor digestive or metabolic processes are no longer eliminated by environmental selection from passing their weaknesses on to succeeding generations. We have learned to compensate. Fortunately, nutritional science has given us methods and products to supplement those natural body processes that nature may have failed to provide in adequate supply.

The Bio-X Diet, if followed, presents total availability of all nutritional needs. There may be individuals, however, whose body mechanisms — for such reasons as age or heredity — lack the ability to obtain complete nutritional value from their food; for them, supplementation is vitally necessary. This is best accomplished with the help of a competent professional nutritionist who can diagnostically evaluate individual dietary needs. Numerous techniques are available to help determine what supplementation may be required.

As a general rule, if nutritional availability is adequate as outlined in the Bio-X Diet, most normal, healthy individuals will require little supplementation during their prime reproductive, child-bearing and raising period — which extends from approximately 15 to 40 years of age. At the end of this period, if longevity and vibrant health are to be maintained, we must actually work against nature. Of course, even during prime years there are circumstances in which supplementation may be required: during pregnancy, for example; or for heavy smoking, excessive stress, lack of energy, sleeplessness, etc. These are examples, incidentally, of instances where advice from a trained nutritionist would be helpful.

In each living plant, animal and human being, there is established at birth a metabolic time clock that guides the individual's growth through infancy and establishes a period of reproduction and maturity. Once the species has procreated itself, nature prepares to eliminate the aging organism to make room for the next generation. Degenerative diseases are a result.

If we intend to lengthen the normal life cycle beyond the reproductive years, there comes a time when we must work against the natural metabolic slowdown which is preparing us for our final recycling.

It has been proven in various races and cultures that proper nutrition, exercise, and freedom from environmental stress can prevent degeneration — and even extend the reproductive years decades beyond what is considered normal in our Euro-American culture. Many experienced nutritionists believe that dietary supplementation, applied as necessary, can play a vital part in increasing the reproductive period; it does so by circumventing, in effect, the time clocks of nature that in later years retard digestive processes.

Dietary supplementation in no way implies ingestion of unnatural substances. It simply brings up to normal requirements the level of digestve fluids, enzymes, vitamins and minerals that various body mechanisms or organs depend upon but may not be producing or metabolizing adequately.

The Bio-X Diet assumes a natural and plentiful supply of vegetables, grains and fruits. There are few geographic areas in Western civilizaton where grains and lentils are not available on a year-around basis. Where such is not the case, supplementation becomes vitally necessary — for example, during certain seasons that may be devoid of fresh produce, or when that which is available has been cultivated in mineral-depleted soil (barren of selenium, for instance).

There has been considerable discussion in recent years concerning megavitamin dosages. The theory seems to be that if a few vitamins are good, a lot of vitamins are better. Under normal health conditions, with a few exceptions, such a belief is erroneous; it can even be dangerous if, in individual or extreme circumstances, it is applied without professional guidance. Oil-soluble vitamins, unbuffered by the balanced ingredients and fiber present in their natural food sources, can potentially be absorbed when taken in excessive amounts and build to highly toxic levels in the liver and fatty tissue.

The majority of vitamins, however, are water-soluble. The body will use what it needs; excesses will simply be excreted. Skeptics will point to our recommendation of bowel tolerance levels of vitamin C as an example of megadosage. Not so. It is only recently that nutritionists, not blinded by orthodoxy, have determined our body's large vitamin C requirements. In previous ages (and even in some present-day primitive cultures) vitamin C was adequately supplied in diets high in green leafy vegetables. As man has evolved in Northern latitudes, this is no longer true.

What we really are recommending is returning to our inherited metabolic requirements. Certain diseases may place extra vitamin or enzyme demand on nutrition. As we have seen, requirements for vitamin A are increased by cancer. What we are discussing here is preventive supplementation for the normal individual. When nutrition is inadequate — or when supplementation is needed to bolster an aging or malfunctioning metabolism — vitamins, enzymes, and other supplements are extremely important additions to dietary intake. However, when synthesized or extracted by man, supplements are, like fiber, second-best to their true food source (assuming the source is available and that sufficient amounts of it can be eaten to fulfill nutritional demand). Excessive supplementation beyond natural need is both expensive and unnecessary.

It may be wise, however, to provide additional nutritional cancer insurance beyond the natural protection provided by the nitriloside foods that are part of the Bio-X Diet — during periods of extended mental or physical stress, for example; or where there is the symptomatic presence of some other metabolic disease which may well be a precursor of cancer, or the individual's family history exhibits an extremely high cancer incidence.

As stated previously, one apricot kernel per each 10 pounds of body weight per day should adequately support the body's intrinsic defense system. If kernels are not available or their bitterness makes them unpalatable, Laevalin tablets taken in professionally recommended amounts would be desirable. The use of only this naturally-extracted amygdalin, as explained in Chapter Nine still applies: 100 mg. to 250 mg. per day will be the ordinarily recommended amount for complete assurance of an actively supported natural immunity from the deadly symptoms of cancer. Additional vitamin A, selenium, or other specifics required for a good cancer-preventive profile, should be determined by your nutrition professional.

Everyone interested in good health should become acquainted with the facilities, products and services provided by local health food stores. Most owners are extremely knowledgeable about nutrition and can be helpful in recommending holistic medical professionals in the community. Based on our experience, this is one field of expertise in which these specialty stores are indispensable — and why they must survive. Not only do they carry a broad selection of health products that are of superior quality, but they are also fully informed about their usage and benefits. All of the products mentioned in this book are available from your holistic physician or health store.

PART 2

The Gourmet Guide
To
Cancer Prevention

The Gourmet Guide to Cancer Prevention

The recipes in our Gourmet Guide to Cancer Prevention have been selected primarily as a guide in returning the unrefined grains and high nitriloside content foods to the diet.

We do not feel it is necessary to include chicken and fish dishes. Recommendations for their preparation abound in the myriad of cookbooks already available. We leave these to the talent and imagination of the cook as we do the preparation of meat dishes, with the reminder that meat should be as lean as possible and when on the menu preferably used as a condiment, casseroled, and extended by the inclusion of vegetables or grains.

Our emphasis here is for palate perfect prevention through pleasing preparation of the high nitriloside foods that have been culturally eliminated from our diets and neglected in even many of the excellent vegetarian cookbooks.

Each sample daily menu contains between three hundred to six hundred milligrams of therapeutic amygdalin which, in most cases, is fifty times the present average adult intake in the United States.

Knowledgeable nutritionists believe that, although many cancer free populations consume larger daily amounts, between 50 mg. and 250 mg. per day of amygdalin should adequately support the body's natural defenses when included with proper enzymes and dietary fiber.

153

Both enzymes and fiber are presented in abundance by the whole grains and lentils in these recipes. This provides the dietary balance which allows inclusion of temperate amounts of processed fats and oils in cooking and for salads and spreads.

Grains and legumes may be purchased in bulk at substantial savings. The Bio-X Diet will result in providential reduction in the food budget while providing a substantial increase in health maintenance.

Search out a greengrocer who can provide fresh organically grown vegetables. While he will, no doubt, include sprouts in his produce, we have included here a brief direction on how to sprout. It is fun, nutritionally enhancing, and as close to having a garden as many urban dwellers can come.

The list of nitriloside plants displays the variety of foods that can provide your natural cancer prevention.

Eating according to your biological experience need not be dull or monotonous.

Get plenty of exercise and, wherever possible, eliminate stress and enjoy your good health.

We hope these sample menus and recipes will guide you to a long active life and... bon appetit!

CHAPTER 13:

A Seven Day Cancer-Free Diet

DAY ONE

Breakfast

-MENU-

Enzyme Cocktail
Millet Crunch Cereal (textured)
with Cashew Nut Milk or Raw Skim Milk
Cereal Blend*
Fruit in Season — Cantaloupe if in Season

* * *

-RECIPE-

Enzyme Cocktail

Papaya juice from the health food store with one tablespoon of 500 Brewers Yeast.

Millet Crunch Cereal

1 c. millet	½ c. wheat germ
½ c. bran	1 T. cinnamon
1 t. salt or kelp	2 c. bottled water
½ c. raisins	Add ⅓ c. flax seed, if desired

1 cup of millet soaked in non-fluoridated water overnight or for 3 or 4 hours. Add the wheat germ, bran, salt, cinnamon and raisins

---

*Many coffee substitutes that are blends of various grains are available at your health food or grocery store.

(and flax seed, if desired) in a baking dish. Barely cover this mixture with the bottled water (approximately 1 cup). Mix together and place in the oven on pilot light until the water has evaporated — leaving cereal moist. Eat while still warm with cashew cream or almond milk or coconut-pineapple juice, tupelo honey, and see how long you feel vital and look good.

Cashew Nut Milk or Cashew Cream

1 c. non-fluoridated water	1 t. honey or 6 to 8 dates
½ c. cashews or blanched almonds or sesame seeds	1 t. vanilla

Wash the unsalted, unroasted raw cashews or almonds thoroughly. Liquefy together in the blender for two to three minutes, adding the honey slowly and 1 t. vanilla.

Lunch

-MENU-

Complete Meal Salad
Bible Bread (available at health food store)
Almond Spread
Fresh Carrot Juice

* * *

-RECIPE-

Complete Meal Salad

Has 542.6 calories, all 8 essential amino acids, 15 grams of protein, rich in vitamins, minerals and enzymes.

½ ripe avocado	2 T. sunflower seeds
7 slices cucumber	½ c. leafy greens
1 c. mung sprouts	⅛ c. salad oil
½ c. summer squash	2 slices tomato or red pepper
1 c. ground apricot kernels	Kelp

Mix together, sprinkle in kelp and pour on the herb dressing.

Herb Dressing

½ t. thyme, ground
1 t. marjoram
½ t. tarragon, ground
½ t. basil, ground
½ c. cold pressed oil

3 T. apple cider vinegar
1 T. finely chopped parsley
½ t. sea salt or 1 t. kelp
1 c. ground apricot kernels

Put in jar and mix together. Pour on your complete salad.

Dinner

-MENU-

Lentil Rice Burgers
Tossed Salad with Herb Dressing
Tropical Cooler Drink
Papaya Leaf Tea
***

-RECIPE-

Lentil Rice Burgers

1 c. dried lentils (2 c. cooked)
1 c. short grain brown rice, raw (2½ - 3 c. cooked)
1 onion, chopped
1 t. sage

Cook lentils and rice separately until done. Drain water off lentils and mash with potato masher. Saute chopped onion in ¼ c. water for about 10 minutes. Combine mashed lentils, rice, onion and sage. Moisten hands and form patties. Bake 325° oven for 30 minutes. Serve with gravy or tomato sauce or in pita bread with tomato and sprouts.

Tossed Salad

(Amount depending on how many servings required)

Romaine lettuce
Red leaf lettuce

Thinly sliced cabbage
Chopped bell pepper

Head lettuce	Alfalfa sprouts
Beet tops	Sunflower seed sprouts
Sliced tomatoes	Raw grated beets
Thinly sliced cauliflower	1 c. slivered apricot kernels
	Herb dressing

Add any small pieces of raw vegetables left over from previous meals and toss with lemon herb dressing. Garnish with sliced radishes and raw mushrooms. Use any of your favorite vegetables as substitutes or additions.

Lemon Herb Dressing

Celery seed to taste	2 sprigs parsley
1 small green onion & tops, chopped very fine	½ t. dried sweet basil
1 t. vegetable broth and seasoning	⅔ c. cold pressed salad oil
	¹⁄₁₆ t. marjoram
½ t. sea salt or 1 t. kelp	Juice of one lemon

Shake vigorously in covered jar until blended. Allow to stand in refrigerator until flavors are blended.

Tropical Cooler Drink

1 banana
1 papaya, cut up
½ c. non-fluoridated water

Pour water in blender; add banana and papaya while blender is in motion. Blend until smooth. Add water, if needed, for desired consistency. Serve in clear glasses or bowls. Makes a delicious enzyme-filled drink. A mango added to the tropical fruit is also delicious in this.

DAY TWO

Breakfast

-MENU-

Glass of Fresh Carrot Juice with Beets
Slenderizing Pancakes with Apricot Sauce
Raw Fruit in Season
Rose Hips Tea with Lemon Juice and Honey
***

-RECIPE-

Pancakes

¼ c. millet	1 t. sea salt or kelp
¼ c. barley	1 t. date spread
¼ c. oats	Lecithin oil
¾ c. raw skim milk	

Soak grains overnight in ¾ c. cold water. Drain water from grains and place in blender with raw skim milk. Whiz 3 to 5 minutes in blender. Add salt, date spread and blend another minute. Continue blending until fluffy and filled with air. Put small amount of lecithin oil in a pan and cook immediately.

Apricot Sauce

2 c. dried apricots	2 oranges
2 c. non-fluoridated water	¾ c. unsweetened pineapple juice

Soak apricots in water overnight. Put apricots, oranges and water in which they were soaked in blender. Whiz briefly. Add pineapple juice slowly while blending.

Lunch

-MENU-

B17 Salad
Raisin Muffin with Date Spread or
Apple Date Spread
Papaya Mint Tea with Honey (unpasteurized) & Lemon
***

-RECIPE-

Glow of Health Salad

½ medium red lettuce
1 c. spinach, pressed firm
Several broccoli tops
Several cauliflower tops
1 stalk sliced celery
4 stalks watercress chopped
½ c. each mung sprouts,
  lentil sprouts, alfalfa
  sprouts

1 small red onion, minced
1 medium cubed tomato
1 large carrot, grated
1 c. cabbage, chopped fine
1 t. sesame seeds
1 c. ground or slivered
  apricot kernels

Dressing

2 T. sesame oil
2 T. lemon juice
1 heaping t. brewers yeast
1 large clove garlic (press
  out and use juice)

½ t. celery seed
½ t. cayenne pepper
½ t. basil

Combine all liquid ingredients in jar. Add yeast and herbs and shake well.

Raisin Muffins

3 c. regular oats
½ c. millet flour
1 c. wheat germ
1 c. bran
⅓ c. sesame seed butter (from health food store)

½ c. raisins
½ t. salt
½ c. ground apricot kernels

Mix all dry ingredients and raisins. Put sesame seed butter in one cup hot water and stir well. Add to the other ingredients and mix well. Let stand 5 to 10 minutes. Pile into prepared muffin pans, bake at 350 degrees until lightly browned about 30 minutes. Or drop by the spoonful on a cookie sheet lightly greased with lecithin oil.

Date Spread

(If you do not care to make this, try a health food store)

1 c. chopped pitted dates	1 c. water

Cook together, stirring often to prevent sticking until dates are very soft. Whiz in blender briefly. Refrigerate. Keeps well for at least one week.

Apple Date Spread

2 chopped apples	½ c. date spread

Whiz in blender until smooth.

Dinner

-MENU-

Fresh Carrot Juice
California Tostada*
Guacamole Dip
Tahini's Purple Surprise Salad
Fresh Pineapple or Papaya
Mint Tea or Papaya Juice

***

-RECIPE-

California Tostada*

4 tortillas	Parsley
Layer of grated lettuce	Cherry tomatoes
Cooked pinto beans	Red chili salsa

Alfalfa sprouts, bean sprouts
Radishes

Taco sauce (if desired)
Guacamole

Lightly fry the corn tortilla in 1 t. olive oil. Put on top of that a layer of grated lettuce. On top of that a layer of cooked pinto beans. On top of that in a circle or kind of a ring, a layer of alfalfa sprouts or mung bean sprouts. Garnish with radishes cut into flowerets, parsley and cherry tomatoes. Top with a large mound of guacamole and red salsa taco sauce if desired.

Guacamole

4 medium avocados, mashed
2 small tomatoes, diced finely
2 green scallions, diced finely
1 to 2 t. of tamari

1 clove garlic, pressed
½ lemon (juiced)
Pinch of cayenne
1 t. olive oil (if desired)

Add mashed avocados and tomatoes and onions together and fold lightly, adding seasoning to taste.

Red Salsa Taco Sauce

2 c. fresh tomatoes (blended)
1 small can peeled green Ortega chilies (or 2 fresh minced & seeded)
1 sweet onion, chopped fine
2 cloves garlic crushed through garlic press

Juice of 2 lemons
1 very ripe avocado, diced finely
1 t. kelp

Blend tomatoes in blender and add remaining ingredients.

Purple Surprise Salad**

1 medium purple cabbage, grated
1 medium purple bermuda onion, sliced thinly
½ c. Fenugreek sprouts

Mix ingredients and toss with lemon herb dressing (recipe above).

---

*California Tostada: Edie May Hunsburger "How I Conquered Cancer Nutritionally"

**Purple Surprise Salad: Tahini Salsbury

DAY THREE

Breakfast

-MENU-

Fresh Squeezed Orange Juice
Millet Cereal, soft and moist, with
raw skim milk (or try apple cider) and
sorghum syrup (an excellent source of B17)

* * *

-RECIPE-

Millet Cereal, Soft and Moist

1 c. whole hulled millet	1 c. raisins
1 qt. non-fluoridated water	½ c. sesame seeds (optional)
1 t. salt	½ c. flax seeds (optional)
1 c. chopped, cored apples	

Put millet, water and salt in a saucepan. Bring to a boil, cover and simmer for 45 minutes or until soft. Remember, never cook on a high heat. Add apples and raisins and sesame seeds. Add sorghum as a sweetener; it is an excellent source of B17. Serve with raw skim milk. Or omit apples and raisins and serve with hot fruit sauce, apricot, apple or berry.

Lunch

-MENU-

Lentil Millet Soup
Sesame Crackers
Devil Tofu

* * *

-RECIPE-

Lentil Millet Soup*

Part I
1 c. millet
1 c. dry lentils
5 c. water
2 t. salt
⅛ t. thyme
⅛ t. oregano

Part II
1 onion, chopped, or 3 grated
  onions
1 grated carrot
¼ c. minced parsley

Cook Part I slowly in a covered pan for 15 minutes. Then combine Part I and Part II. Add 1 or 2 chopped tomatoes or small can whole tomatoes. Simmer all ingredients together 45 minutes or until lentils and millet are tender. Add more water if needed.

Sesame Crackers

⅓ c. macadamia nuts (an excellent sourse of B17)
⅓ c. sesame seeds

Grind macadamia nuts and sesame seeds separately until slightly pasty. Put into blender and add ⅔ cup water. Blend until smooth.

Put the following in a bowl and mix well:

½ c. millet
½ c. barley flour
¼ c. rye flour

½ c. wheat germ
½ t. salt
⅓ c. full fat soy flour, sifted

Add blended mixture to dry ingredients. Mix well and knead lightly. Dough should not be sticky when all dry ingredients are kneaded in. If sticky, add a bit more flour as needed. Roll between waxed paper until very thin, ⅛" or less. Put on a cookie sheet that has been prepared with a thin film of lecithin oil. Cut in squares and prick with a fork. Bake at 400 degrees until lightly brown and crisp. Walnuts, pecans or cashews can be substituted for macadamia nuts but macadamia nuts are the highest in B17.

Note: Crackers at edges of pan will brown first. Remove these and continue the rest until done.

---

*B17 natural sources

Tahini* Devil Tofu

2 pkgs. Tofu
¼ bunch celery, diced
8 finely chopped green onions
1 c. eggless mayonnaise to
　desired consistency
½ t. dried mustard, to taste

½ c. or juice of 1 lemon
2 T. tumeric to desired color
　(it should look about the color
　of egg yolk)
2 T. tamari
Pinch sea salt or Spike to taste

Mash tofu and mix ingredients. To decorate, form in the shape of a pineapple in a mold. Shape mixture in loaf of oval size on platter. Place pineapple leaves at top. Arrange pimento criss-crossed across the top to form squares. Fill squares with diced round olives. Serve with sesame crackers for hors d'oeuvres.

Dinner

-MENU-

Liver Athens (for liver haters)
Gazpacho
Uncooked Applesauce
Spinach Mushroom Salad (See Chapter 15)
Cinnamon Orange Tea with Lemon and Honey
(unpasteurized if desired)

* * *

-RECIPE-
Liver Athens

4 large onions
½ t. vegetable salt
Pinch of cayenne pepper
1 t. vegetable oil, cold
　pressed
Sesame oil or olive oil

1 lb. calf liver or baby
　beef liver
½ c. wheat germ**
½ c. whole-wheat flour
2 c. fresh mushrooms

Saute onions until transparent. Slice liver into small strips 2″ by

---

*Tahini Salsbury
**Wheat germ becomes rancid quickly. Rancid oil has been found to be a major cause of aging. Therefore, when possible buy your wheat germ canned or frozen, or keep it in the freezer.

¼″ thick, discarding skin and veins. In dish or plastic bag combine wheat germ, whole-wheat flour, vegetable salt, cayenne. Coat strips of liver in this mixture and saute lightly rotating until all surfaces of liver are lightly browned. Combine mushrooms in pan with liver; saute lightly. Do not overcook liver. *Serves 6.*

Uncooked Applesauce

3 organic sweet apples
½ c. water
Honey (if desired)

Cut up the apples (peels, cores, seeds and all). Pour ½ c. of water into the blender. Drop in the cut-up apples. Do not blend too long or they will oxidize. Eat right away.

Gazpacho
(A chilled Mexican soup)

Fresh tomatoes
1 large cucumber
1 large onion (peeled or
   green)
1 bell pepper
1 can pimento

¼ c. apple cider vinegar
1 chile pepper
Kelp
Garlic (chopped fine)
Vegetable seasoning
1 can sliced ripe olives

Put tomatoes in blender and puree to make about 18 or 20 oz. Cut onion and pepper into cubes. Put in blender. Add pimento, kelp, garlic, seasoning, oil and vinegar. Puree. Chill at least 3 hours. Also chill at least six serving bowls and a soup tureen. Chop fresh tomato, cucumber, onion, green pepper. Place in separate bowls. Chill olives in small bowl, sprinkle over top of each serving.

###

DAY FOUR

Breakfast

-MENU-

Fresh Carrot Juice
Fruit in Season
Millet soy waffles covered in berry
sauce or fruit spread
Brigham or Mormon Tea to top it off

***

-RECIPE-

Millet Soy Waffles

2 ¼ c. water, non-fluoridated
1 ¼ c. millet flour or 1 c.
millet seeds
½ t. salt

1 c. soaked soy beans
(equivalent of ½ c. dry)

Soak beans several hours or overnight in sufficient water to keep covered. Drain. Discard water (soaked, drained soy beans may be kept in refrigerator for a week or a freezer for longer periods; keep on hand for immediate use).

Combine all ingredients and blend until light and foamy, about ½ minute. Let stand while waffle iron is heating. The batter thickens on standing. Blend briefly. Pour into pitcher for convenience. Bake in hot iron for 8 minutes or until brown. If you do not wish to use the oil you may put sesame seeds in the waffle iron — the oil from the sesame seeds will grease the waffle iron and keep it from sticking. Set timer for 8 minutes and do not open before time is up. Cook a few seconds longer if the iron sticks. When serving a large number bake waffles ahead. Cook, stack and cover with wax paper. Just before serving, reheat in waffle iron, oven or toaster briefly. These can be frozen nicely.

Berry Sauce

4 c. frozen, unsweetened berries, thawed

2 t. tapioca, ground

Juice & water to make 1 ½ c. liquid

1 to 2 very ripe bananas

Pour juice over berries into two cup measure. Add water to make 1½ cups and put in blender. Add bananas and tapioca. Whiz briefly. Place in saucepan and cook over medium heat until thickened. Add berries and heat through.

Fruit Spread

1 each orange, yellow apple, banana

Blend together until smooth. Refrigerate. Will keep well one or two days.

Lunch

-MENU-

Lentil Millet Soup

Sesame Crackers

Sprout Salad

Chamomile Tea with Honey (unpasteurized)
and lemon if desired

***

-RECIPE-

Lentil Millet Soup

Part I

1 c. millet

1 c. dry lentils

5 c. water

2 t. salt

⅛ t. thyme

⅛ t. oregano

Part II

1 onion, chopped or 3 green onions

1 grated carrot

¼ c. minced parsley

Cook Part I slowly in separate covered pan for 15 minutes. Then combine Parts I and II. Add one or two chopped tomatoes or small whole tomatoes. Simmer ingredients together for 45 minutes or until lentils and millet are tender. Add more water if needed.

Sesame Crackers

(See page 164)

(Lentil Millet Soup also on page 164)

Sprout Salad

2 c. bean sprouts	½ c. raw fresh peas
2 c. alfalfa sprouts	8 dates, pitted and chopped
1 c. raw mushrooms, sliced	Avocado dressing

Mix in large bowl and top each serving with avocado dressing. Or, for individual salads serve on lettuce leaf with dressing. Or, cupped in red cabbage leaves.

Avocado Dressing

1 large ripe avocado	½ t. salt
2 T. lemon juice	2 T. mayonnaise
2 T. minced onion	Pinch of salt
2 T. chopped pimento or red bell pepper	

Mash avocado with fork. Add rest of ingredients.

Dinner

-MENU-

Harvest Stew served over Millet & Brown Rice
Fruit Kabob for Dessert (See page 178 under day 6)
Sparkling Cider as a Beverage
***

-RECIPE-

Harvest Stew

½ head cabbage	1 t. Worcestershire
4 zucchini squash	½ t. sesame oil
1 onion	1 c. mushrooms
1 c. pumpkin seeds	Vegasal to taste

Saute onions until translucent; then put in the zucchini, cabbage, mushrooms and remaining ingredients. Season with Vegasal and while it is cooking slowly on a very, very low heat add V-8 juice to the vegetables. Add Worcestershire. Just before serving, add 1 cup of pumpkin seeds for that crisp texture. Serve over a bed of ½ millet, ½ brown rice. Remember to cook this on a very low heat to protect the enzymes.

DAY FIVE

Breakfast

-MENU-

Fresh Carrot Juice
Old Fashioned Buckweat Cakes
Fruit in Season
Cup of piping hot Split Pea Soup
(why not soup for breakfast!)

***

-RECIPE-

Old Fashioned Buckwheat Cakes

1½ c. buckwheat flour
½ c. whole wheat flour
1 T. sorghum or honey
1 t. sea salt

1 t. baking powder
1 T. safflower or sesame oil
1½ c. spring water
1 egg white

In a large bowl stir dry ingredients. Add oil, sorghum and water, then beaten egg white, a little at a time as you mix. Pour small amount onto a hot oiled griddle or skillet. Turn cakes when bubbles appear. Serve hot with sorghum maple syrup.

Sorghum Maple Syrup

Combine ¼ cup maple syrup with 2 T. sorghum, ¼ cup water and heat over low flame. Serve hot over Buckwheat Cakes.

Split Pea Soup

1 lb. split peas covered with two inches of water. Add 2 diced carrots, 1 chopped onion, 2 stalks celery chopped, 1 t. celery or vegetable salt. Cook until tender — stir often. Blend for smooth soup or serve as is, with garlic toast or zwieback.

Lunch

-MENU-

Stuffed Red Bell Pepper
Potato Salad
Millet Chews for Dessert
with Sesame Butter Spread

* * *

-RECIPE-

Stuffed Red Bell Peppers

Use small red bell peppers, because the red have more vitamin C. Cut off top and scoop out seeds. Fill with the following: fine chopped cabbage, green onions, finely chopped parsley, dill weed and mayonnaise (eggless, of course). Mix together and fill peppers. This is also a good sandwich filling.

Potato Salad

2 qts. cooked potatoes	¼ c. chopped onion
½ c. chopped celery	2 T. chopped pimento
½ c. shredded carrot	1 c. eggless mayonnaise
½ c. chopped bell pepper	¼ c. lemon juice
(green to give a contrast to	1 t. salt
the red)	½ t. paprika

Dice and salt potatoes. Mix with celery, carrot, bell pepper, onion and pimento. Serve potato salad from an ice cream scoop on a fresh leaf of green lettuce or kale.

B17 Millet Chews

These are great for the children's lunches, backpacks, etc.

1 c. cooked millet
1½ c. date pieces, finely chopped
½ c. coconut, shredded
1 c. nut butter of choice
½ c. sorghum
½ c. sesame seeds

1 t. vanilla

2 T. orange rind, finely grated (from fresh, hopefully organically grown oranges)*

1 T. lemon rind (from fresh organically grown lemons)*

½ t. sea salt

Mix all ingredients well. Use long wooden spoon and plenty of elbow grease. You may find it easier and preferable to mix the candy with your hands. Shape into two inch long rolls the thickness of your thumb, wrap in wax paper and chill until hard.

Dinner

-MENU-

Sweet Potato Pie
Garbanzo Lima Salad
Pumpkin Pie
Cereal Blend with Honey (if desired)

* * *

-RECIPE-

Sweet Potato Pie

Boil and mash 3 lbs. sweet potatoes. One large can of sweet potatoes, for convenience sake, equals 2 lbs. Blend in 3 well-beaten egg yolks, 1 T. melted butter, 1 t. salt, 1 cup raw skim milk for thicker texture. Blend all this together; fold in 3 well-beaten egg whites. Butter ring mold or put in buttered dish. Sprinkle with slivered macadamia nuts.

Pumpkin Pie in Granola Crust

1½ c. pumpkin or squash	½ c. soy or raw skim milk
2 T. honey	½ t. vanilla
¼ c. date sugar	½ t. lemon rind or extract
3 T. Arrowroot powder	1 t. coriander seed, ground
¼ t. salt	

---

*Commercial citrus rinds may be toxic.

Mix ingredients in saucepan and cook until thick, stirring occasionally. Put into blender and whiz until smooth. Pour into baked pie shell. Refrigerate until ready to serve.

Granola Pie Crust

1½ c. coconut
1½ c. granola (blended fine in the blender)
1 c. almonds or macadamia nuts (or ½ each), ground in blender
¼ c. whole wheat flour or whole wheat pastry flour
¼ c. wheat germ
1 t. vanilla
½ to ⅔ c. raw skim or soy milk or water

Mix ingredients together in a bowl with spoon. Then press into pie pan using spoon. Bake at 350 degrees for about 8 to 10 minutes. Watch carefully to prevent burning.

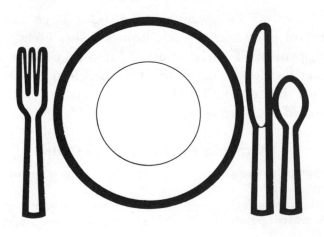

DAY SIX

Breakfast

-MENU-

Fresh Carrot & Beet Juice
Pot of Lentils
(another piping hot delicious soup for breakfast)
Honeydew Melon or Fruit in Season
Mint Tea

***

-RECIPE-

Pot of Lentils

2 c. uncooked lentils
1 chopped onion
1 chopped carrot
½ c. chopped celery
¼ c. chopped bell pepper
2 T. vegetable seasoning

1 can tomato soup or tomato paste
½ t. oregano
1 t. cumin
1 t. salt

Cook lentils, onion, carrot, celery and bell pepper together in 4 cups of water. Add other ingredients; simmer until done.

Lunch

-MENU-

Millet and Brown Rice Combo
Spinach and Mushroom Salad
Savory Garbanzos

***

-RECIPE-

Method of preparation for Millet and Brown Rice — see page 210. However, add soy sauce to the water in which you cook the millet and brown rice.

Savory Garbanzos

3 c. garbanzos, cooked (refer to p. 229)
½ bell pepper, minced
¼ t. sweet basil
1 onion, minced
2 c. canned tomatoes

Combine all ingredients and pour into a casserole. Bake at 350 degrees for 25 to 30 minutes, adding a little water if necessary. Serves 6 to 8.

Dinner

-MENU-

Impressive Company Dinner
Dairyless Spanakopita or Greek Spinach Pie
(a dish so light and delicious the Greeks,
who know fine food, have made it a tradition)
Tahini's Taboole
Fruit Kabobs
Cider Ale (we, of course, know it is best to
drink the beverage an hour before the meal). Cider
ale is a lovely company treat; non-alcoholic, of course.

* * *

-RECIPE-

Spanakopita

Filo dough (found at gourmet food markets)
Soy margarine (health food store)
¼ t. thyme
Spinach
Mushrooms, sliced

1 lb. feta cheese or tofu (for those who want to avoid dairy products)
Sea Salt, ¼ t. or to taste
¼ t. basil
¼ t. coriander

Onions
Nutmeg

Brush 2 layers of filo dough in melted soy margarine. If you are having a hard time keeping the filo dough from breaking, put it in your freezer while you prepare the other ingredients. Saute onions until translucent in soy margarine or butter. Add mushrooms. Bring water to boil. Put spinach and 1 t. nutmeg in the water. Take off the stove while semi-cooked. Dice spinach fine, then mix with other ingredients and spices. Marinate feta cheese or tofu in nutmeg water or cider vinegar with coriander and basil. Mash feta cheese or tofu with onions, mushrooms, spinach. Place in double layer of brushed filo and roll. Place more in and roll until you have a spinach-filled roll that is a taste delight.

Tahini's Taboole

2 cucumbers
1 bunch parsley
1 head lettuce
6 tomatoes
4 green scallions

2½ c. sprouted wheat berries, from health food store. Cover with water for approximately 3 days until sprouted.

Mix all ingredients except sprouted berries. Add berries. Use garlic lemon dressing.

Garlic Lemon Dressing

2 cups olive oil
1 to 10 cloves garlic buds, blended in blender

1 c. lemon juice
Vegasal to taste

Mix all together and garnish around the sides of the bowl with parsley.

Fruit Kabobs

If you can get fresh pineapple, fresh strawberries and fresh papaya, buy some bamboo skewers approximately 7 inches long, usually available at your hardware store. Cut the pineapple and papaya in chunks. Put a chunk of pineapple on the skewer; next a bright, red strawberry; next a chunk of papaya until you have covered skewer, leaving a small handle to pick up with. Serve with a small dish of whipped nut cream to dip the fruit in, fondue style. This is a lovely company dish. Many times if you just put a large bowl of the whipped nut cream in the middle of the table, it encourages your guests to "loosen up" because they all have to share the same bowl. Also, these can be served with the chunks of fruit in a bowl with enough skewers so that guests can dip one piece of fruit at a time into the nut cream. This is a festive, beautiful and tasty meal.

DAY SEVEN

Breakfast

-MENU-

Fresh Carrot Juice
Scrambled Tofu
Lentil Millet Patties with Tomato Sauce
Juniper Berry Tea or Burdock Tea
(a good blood purifier)

***

-RECIPE-

Scrambled Tofu

1 block tofu (available at fine food stores everywhere)
2 T. soy sauce
⅛ t. turmeric
1-1½ t. chicken-like seasoning (Loma Linda's Savorex has a natural nutritious flavoring that is available at your health food store)
1 bunch green onions with tops

Drain the tofu well, then cube it. Brown. Add soy sauce, chopped onions and seasonings. Continue cooking and scrambling until onions are done.

Lentil Millet Patties

Can be fixed the night before and heated at a very low heat in the oven with the tomato sauce.

1 c. dried lentils, picked over and washed	2 eggs lightly beaten
Water	Wheat germ
¾ c. whole hulled millet	Sesame oil for frying
1 onion, chopped	(Recipe for tomato sauce to follow)
Sea salt and cayenne	
Pepper to taste (optional)	

Put lentils in a saucepan with water to cover, bring to a boil and cook until tender, simmering about 45 minutes. Put millet and 1½ cups water in a second sauce pan. Cover and simmer 30 minutes or until tender and water is absorbed. Drain the lentils and mix with millet. Add onion, sea salt or Vegasal and cayenne. Shape mixture into patties. Dip into beaten egg and then into wheat germ. Heat sesame or olive oil in heavy skillet and fry patties in it until golden. Drain on paper towels and serve with tomato sauce. Serves 6.

Tomato Sauce

12 large ripe tomatoes, skinned and chopped	6 stalks of celery, diced
2 green peppers, seeded	2 T. fresh chives
2 onions, chopped	2 T. chopped fresh parsley
2 carrots, chopped	2 T. chopped fresh basil
	2 cloves garlic finely chopped

Combine all ingredients in a stainless steel or porcelainized steel pan or casserole. Bring to a boil and simmer uncovered for 45 minutes. Puree in a blender if desired. Refrigerate overnight or freeze for future use if desired. Yield about 2 quarts.

Lunch

-MENU-

Meatless Burger (watch out McDonalds!)

***

-RECIPE-

Meatless Burger

Saute in a bit of water: 1½ onions chopped fine, ½ lb. mushrooms chopped fine, 1 T. sweet basil, 1 T. chopped garlic, 1 T. garlic powder or ½ T. garlic powder to taste, ¼ c. chicken-like seasoning (Savorex from health food store), 1½ t. Dr. Bronner's (a health food store type of bouillon with vitamins and minerals). Cook until well done in just enough water to cover azuki beans, ¾ c.

lentils. Bring ¾ c. water to boil and ¼ c. bulgar wheat. Remove from heat. Let absorb moisture. Add 1½ c. rolled oats, 1¼ c. wheat germ, ¼ c. sesame seeds or sunflower seeds, ¼ c. macademia nuts chopped. Mix all together well. Form into patties. This may be frozen and when thawed add wheat germ, millet or potato flour to thicken if necessary. Saute or broil. This makes a great hamburger substitute between two pieces of mixed grain bread and eggless mayonnaise and energy spread.

Energy Spread

1 c. mayonnaise	2 T. brewer's yeast
½ t. turmeric	¼ t. soy sauce

Mix, chill and let stand 2 hours before serving on bread, toast or baked potatoes.

Dinner

-MENU-

Ratatouilli
Cucumber Salad with Dressing
Bread
Lemon Pie

***

-RECIPE-

Ratatouilli

1 medium onion chopped	2 c. stewed tomatoes
1 glove garlic, minced	1 t. dried basil
2 zucchini squash thinly sliced	1 T. flaked dry parsley
1 small eggplant peeled and cubed	1 t. sea salt or Vegasal
1 bell pepper cut into 1″ pieces	1 t. Worcestershire

Saute onions and garlic for five minutes. Add squash, eggplant and bell pepper to skillet and cook for 10 minutes more, stirring gently. Add small amount of water if needed. Stir in tomatoes and seasoning. Reduce heat to low, cover skillet tightly and cook 15 minutes more. Serve immediately over a mixture of one-half cooked millet and one-half cooked brown rice (cooked in water with 1 T. soy sauce added).

CHAPTER 14:

The Children's Lunch Box

LUNCH BOX SUGGESTIONS OR SCHOOL LUNCHES

The number one killer of children under 14 years old is cancer.* There is no sadder lament than to see a child seemingly eaten away by this voracious killer. Life comes from life and so we want to include in our loved ones' lunches as much live food as possible. We want well balanced meals for growing children for whom optimum nutrition is so important.

Many different B-17 enzyme foods can be included such as hearty soup (millet), dried fruits wrapped around apricot kernels, baked beans, raw vegetable sticks, nuts, seeds and granola. A plastic thermos is a necessity for many of these variations. I instituted what I considered an insurance policy against the loss of a thermos bottle and lunch swapping which also lets he or she know mother was thinking of them as they enjoyed their lunch.

Lunch box surprises for the school lunch

1. A note from mother in which I complimented my child on something — even if it was the way his or her arm hung from its socket. The children loved the compliments (of course, they are only little people after all) but were in mortal fear of their school mates seeing it.

2. A new pencil or eraser.

3. A prize similar to an item stuffed in their Christmas stocking.

---

*According to the A.C.S. fact book

4. A surprise apple. Remove core, stuff raisins, dates and a rolled up note with a funny line such as "Dear Teacher: Please do not hit Sean — we only hit him in self-defense."

5. A greeting card. A Christmas card in April imploring them not to open until Christmas.

6. Now you think of some!

Lentil Soup Recipe #2
(one given previously in 7-day plan)

4 c. stock or water
1 c. dried lentils, washed
1 large white onion, diced
2 stalks celery plus tops, chopped
½ green bell pepper, diced
2 medium carrots
1 t. cumin
1 t. nutmeg
1 t. cayenne pepper (optional)
1 t. celery seed
1 T. tamari soy sauce
1 t. thyme
1 bay leaf (remove before serving)
Few sprigs of parsley
1 t. sweet basil

Bring liquid to a boil and add the lentils. Reduce heat and simmer for 30 minutes, partially covered. Add remainder of ingredients and simmer for 20 minutes more. Add 1 T. of tamari last (more or less to taste) to preserve its nutritional content. Remove half of soup from pan to blender and whiz for a few seconds to obtain a thick, warm lentil puree. Mix back into the remaning soup in the pot, stir to desired consistency. Top with minced parsley and put in the thermos.

Magical Millet Soup

2 qt. stock, liquid or water
¾ c. uncooked millet
2 c. zucchini squash, sliced
1 large onion, diced (red onions have a mellower flavor and are preferred)
2 stalks celery, w/tops, chopped
1 c. small mushrooms (wash and leave whole)
1 t. basil
½ t. thyme
1 t. dried mint
½ c. parsley, finely chopped
juice of 1 lemon

Bring stock or water to boil in a large pot. Then add millet, onion and celery. Simmer gently in covered pot 30 to 40 minutes.

During the last 10 minutes of cooking add remainder of ingredients.

Black-eyed Pea Soup

Black-eyed peas, of course, are a rich source of B-17

2 c. black-eyed peas, cooked
2 stalks celery, chopped
3 c. vegetable stock (stock that you cook the peas in)
2 T. Vegasal or other seasoning
1 bunch (about 4) leaks (if desired), chopped fine
4 T. sesame oil
1 c. raw skimmed milk
½ t. cayenne pepper
1 T. sorghum

In a soup pot add chopped leaks (tops included), celery and oil. Cook 10 minutes stirring occasionally. Add black-eyed peas, stock and vegetable seasoning. Stir, cover and cook on low heat 15 minutes. Add milk, sorghum, cayenne and more seasoning according to taste. Stir and simmer 10 more minutes. Serve garnished with chopped watercress.

Of course, do not forget the lentil millet soup given in the 7-day lunch, p. 164, served with sesame crackers.

Hearty Vegetable Soup

2 qts. water
4 T. vegetable or chicken-like seasoning
1 large beet, grated
1 large onion, chopped
2 to 3 diced carrots
1 large potato, cubed
1 pkg. frozen green beans
2 cups garden peas
1 pkg. frozen or fresh zucchini, sliced
Chopped greens — cabbage, chard, etc.
2 large tomatoes, chopped
1 can garbanzos
½ c. barley
Herbs to season
3 bay leaves
dill weed, thyme, sweet basil, rosemary, marjoram, garlic powder
sea salt to taste

Cook barley 30 minutes in 2 qts. water. Add rest of ingredients and simmer slowly on low heat until tender. Can vary vegetables to suit taste.

Minestrone Soup

Bring 3 qts. water to a boil in large pot. Add 2 cups millet. Add 2 to 3 cups chopped vegetables — equal amounts of celery, cabbage, chard, onions, carrots, etc. Add: 4-5 T. tomato sauce or 2 fresh tomatoes chopped, 1 clove garlic mashed, salt to taste, Spike or Vegasal. Cook for at least one hour. For last ½ hour add the vegetable or amino acid pasta you wish. Meanwhile cook 1 cup of lima beans (for faster cooking soak overnight). When beans are done, blend and add e soup when it is done. If you cook soup after adding beans, be sure to stir often to prevent burning.

Black Bean Soup

Saute in ½ cup of water 1 sliced onion and 1 clove garlic minced. Add black beans and 2 cups of black-eyed peas, soaked. Cover with water and cook for ½ hour. Add more water as needed. Add 1 bay leaf, 1 T. oregano, 4 T. Dr. Bronner's (bouillon-like substance rich in vitamins and minerals that you can get at your health food store), 3 T. chicken-like seasoning, 1 qt. canned tomatoes cut in pieces, 1 qt. tomato sauce, Vegasal or Spike as needed. Add 2 cups zucchini sliced in circles, 1½ cup bell pepper cut in medium pieces, 5 t. lemon juice (approx.). Cook until done. Add ½ cup minced parsley near end of cooking period and finish cooking. Add more water if needed, to make soupy consistency.

Cream of Carrot Soup

Saute in ¼ cup water 1 large onion sliced thin, 1 T. fresh minced garlic. Add 1 cup fresh whole mushrooms, 6 carrots washed and peeled. Cover with hot water about 3 inches above vegetables and cook until tender. Remove from heat and cool slightly. Blend in blender with ⅓ cup corn starch, 1 T. sweet basil, ½ t. tarragon, 3 T. chicken seasoning (Savorex), ¼ cup millet flour, ½ t. chervil, 1 T. Magi, 1 T. Dr. Bronner's. Return to large soup pot and add 1 to 2 t. lemon juice, ½ cup white grape juice (Lehr's or Carmel). Bring just to a boil and let simmer. Stir, turn off heat and add 2 cups of raw skimmed milk.

SANDWICHES AND SANDWICH FILLINGS

Quickie Bean Sandwich

Fill in with any kind of bean that has B-17 in it — either broad beans, chick peas, garbanzos, fava, kidney, lentils sprouted, limas, mung, navy or scarlet runners can be used in this recipe so you can use a variety of baked beans that have B-17.

Whole wheat bread slices	Tomatoes (sliced)
Bean of your choice (baked)	Pimento cashew sauce

Spoon bean of your choice onto the bread. Lay slice of tomato on top of the beans. Top with pimento cashew sauce. Put in 200 degree oven until heated, about 10 minutes.

Pimento Cashew Sauce

4 c. water	1¼ T. onion powder
4 c. cashews	1¼ T. garlic powder
1¼ t. salt	12 T. brewers yeast flakes
1⅓ c. lemon juice	(¾ cup)
16 oz. pimento	

Whiz all together, except lemon juice. Then add lemon juice while blending.

This can take the place of peanut butter and is far more nutritious.

Savory Garbanzo Sandwich Filling

1 c. dry garbanzos, soaked	2 T. nut milk
3 green onions	Sesame seeds
1 to 2 cloves garlic (optional)	Salt to taste or kelp
⅓ c. parsley sprigs, packed	Cumin, to taste

Drain beans and put through fine blade of meat grinder with onions, parsley and garlic. Mix well. Add milk and seasonings. Let stand 15 minutes or so. Mixture will be soft. Saute in frying pan, tossing and turning with spatula. Add a bit of water if needed.

Lima Bean Filling

Mash two cups cooked lima beans or canned. Saute 1 cup onion, chopped fine, 2 cloves garlic, minced bacon bits (optional) — the soy imitation bacon bits, of course, are best. Mix with beans along with 1 t. oregano, ¾ c. mayonnaise, salt to taste, 1 T. soy sauce, wheat germ to thicken.

Carrot Macadamian Filling

1 c. finely grated carrots
½ c. chopped macadamia nuts
  (or cashews)

¼ c. mayonnaise
1 t. salt
1 t. lemon juice

Combine all ingredients. Chill. Yield about 1½ cups.

Garbanzo Sandwich Filling

1 can garbanzos, 15 oz.
1 can olives, 6 oz., drained
½ small onion

Grind the above with the finest blade of meat grinder. Mix mixture in skillet and add ½ t. Vegex or 1 t. soy sauce and 1 T. brewers yeast mixed together. Stir and saute for a few minutes. Serve as is or mix with mayonnaise for a sandwich spread or to put on toast.

Basic Nut Butter

Place 1½ cups whole or broken nuts in blender. Blend until fine and then add water in the amounts listed below depending on the type of nuts used. Add a small amount of water at a time blending after each addition. Start and stop as necessary. Use a spatula to keep butter in motion. Mixture is thick — to avoid overtaxing the motor make nut butter in small batches. Add salt to taste. Whiz until very smooth. Makes about 1 cup.

Almonds, blanched - 2 to 3 T.
Cashews, toasted   - 4 to 6 T.
Peanuts, toasted   - 2 to 4 T.
Pecans   - 1½ T.
Pine nuts   - 1 to 2 T.

Spread whole wheat bread with any one of your basic nut butters, add sliced bananas and raisins to the top.

Olive Sandwich Filling

1 c. chopped ripe olives

½ c. chopped macadamia nuts

¼ c. almonds, chopped fine

¼ c. sesame or sunflower seeds

¼ c. celery, chopped fine

Mix with enough mayonnaise to moisten.

Eggless Burgers

1 t. Savorex or Vegex

¼ c. hot water

1 c. grated raw potatoes

1 c. oatmeal

½ c. onion, chopped fine

¼ c. chopped macadamia nuts

⅓ c. celery, chopped fine

1 sprig parsley, chopped

1 c. millet

2 T. chopped olives

1 T. wheat germ

⅛ t. sage

1 t. garlic salt

1 t. soy sauce

¼ t. salt or to taste

Dissolve Savorex in hot water. Mix all ingredients together and form into patties. If batter is too thick, add more water. Saute slowly or broil.

Bean Burgers

2 cups cooked beans (picked from the list of B-17 beans on p. 229, either black eyed, broad, chick peas, garbanzos, kidney, lentils, lima, mung, navy, peas or scarlet runners

⅔ c. ground sunflower seeds

¼ c. chopped onion

¼ t. cumin

1 t. Vegasal, Spike or sea salt

3 to 4 T. catsup or tomato sauce

½ c. wheat germ

Combine all ingredients adding enough wheat germ so mixture will hold its shape. Form 8 patties and bake at 200° for 45 minutes or if you are in a hurry bake at 350° for 15 to 20 minutes. Or broil 5 minutes on each side until lightly browned and crusty.

Note: 1 cup dry beans cooks up to 3 cups.

Soy Spread

⅓ cup soy flour, ⅓ cup millet flour (low heat, 300 degrees). Let cool. Mix with 1¾ cup water. Cool by stirring constantly about 3 minutes. Reduce heat to a simmer and cook 10 minutes. Add ½ t. salt, 2 T. lemon juice, ¼ t. garlic powder, 1 t. honey. Stir well, refrigerate. Keeps up to two weeks. Whip with a fork to smooth before serving. (May have to add water if it is too thick). May be used as a sandwich spread or mayonnaise.

Tofu Dressing

Tofu   Onion powder to taste
Raw skimmed milk

Use enough raw skimmed milk to blend with tofu to make a creamy consistency. This has very little taste of its own — season to your own taste.

California Mission Sandwich

Into a corn tortilla or Bible bread bought at the health food store (if you use Bible bread slit it open and stuff the Bible bread, otherwise a corn tortilla without preservatives). Mash avocado or slice and season with kelp, vegetable seasoning and lemon juice. Warm tortilla or bread. If using Bible bread, split the loaf and spread each side with eggless mayonnaise. Spread with avocado. Add hot chili peppers or sweet bell peppers or both, depending upon your taste. Add raw mushroom slices and sprinkle with sunflower seeds. Top with alfalfa sprouts, a good covering. I serve them open face at home, but put the second slice on top for a lunch box or brown bag lunch.

Nut Loaf

1 c. carrots   1 c. tomatoes
½ c. chopped parsley   ½ c. bell pepper pieces
1 clove garlic, optional   2 T. oil
Ground nuts   Favorite herb (sage or dill)

Put all through a grinder, mix and pack into a loaf pan to serve or make sandwich.

Avocado Spread

This can be put inside of Bible bread or inside of a corn tortilla as a luncheon treat.

2 avocados, mashed
2 T. lemon juice
2 T. mayonnaise

1 T. grated onion
½ t. salt, or to taste

Mix all ingredients well. Chill. Yield about 1 cup.

CHAPTER 15:

Salads, Salad Dressings, Spreads and Sauces

Hawaiian Carrot Salad

Toss together the following:

Grated carrots
Grated coconut
Grated red apples and/or pineapple tidbits
Raisins or currants
Cashews or macadamia nuts

You may use mayonnaise to moisten or serve with whipped nut cream as a garnish.

Vitamin Salad

Serve mounds of seasoned cabbage slaw, shredded beets and shredded carrots on lettuce leaf or leaves of a red cabbage. In balls they make a beautiful display.

Stuffed Tomato Salad

Core tomatoes and cut diagonally into 6 or 8 sections almost through, leaving sections connected at base. Spread to look like flowers and place on crisp greens. Stuff with tofu cottage cheese. Or in tiny tomatoes individually stuffed as an hors d'oeuvre.

Tofu Cottage Cheese

½ c. tofu
¼ t. celery salt
¼ t. onion powder or chopped
  green onions

Pinch of garlic salt
¼ t. soy sauce

Mix together with fork to medium curds. Fill tomatoes and garnish with pimento and green pepper. Season to taste. Use an ice cream scoop and put on top of sliced tomato with a sprig of parsley.

Stuffed Avocado Salad

Peel desired amount of avocados. Cut in half and remove seeds. Fill with the following:

Finely diced green beans	Fresh cauliflower
Diced celery	Beets cut in small pieces
Chopped onion	

Mix together with a small amount of mayonnaise and fill avocado halves.

Watercress Bean Sprout Salad

Watercress and any of the sprouts rich in B-17: alfalfa, bamboo, fava, garbanzo, mung, wheat berry sprouts.

Combine bean sprouts, green onion, celery and water chestnuts. Mix with a salad dressing and serve on a bed of watercress.

Stuffed Tomatoes

Scoop the pulp from the inside of four tomatoes. Drain off juice and put pulp in bowl. Add mayonnaise, minced parsley, any of the B-17 sprouts and ground pecans or sunflower seed meal to pulp. Add together and fill tomatoes. Garnish with a sprig of parsley. Save tomato juice to use in soup.

Hors d'oeuvre Salad

Celery sticks	Sliced turnips
Carrot sticks	Sliced beets
Zucchini sticks	Raw broccoli slices
Cherry tomatoes	Mushrooms
Radishes	Cauliflower

Serve on a large round platter. Arrange in 8 sections around the outside of the platter. Set a dish of guacamole dip in the center and see your friends devour this one.

Liquid Salad in a Glass

¾ c. finely chopped onion
¾ t. minced garlic
1½ c. bell pepper, finely chopped
3½ c. fresh tomatoes, diced
1 T. paprika
1 T. olive oil

½ c. fresh lemon juice
1 c. water
½ c. thinly sliced
cucumbers
1 T. kelp

Blend and chill 2 to 3 hours. Add cucumber just before serving.

Sprout Salad

1 c. of your favorite sprouts
½ c. grated celery
½ c. diced onions
½ c. grated onions
1 diced red pepper
Leaf lettuce

Avocado
Tomato
Lemon juice
Kelp
Vegetable seasoning

Combine the sprouts, celery, onions and red pepper. Mix thoroughly in a large bowl. Toss with lemon juice, kelp and vegetable seasoning. Serve on a leaf of lettuce or on a leaf of red cabbage and garnish with avocado and tomato.

Cauliflower Salad

Raw cauliflowerets, sliced
Chopped bell peppers
Chopped carrots

Watercress or parsley
Eggless mayonnaise

Mix all ingredients with eggless mayonnaise and serve on a bed of greens.

Super Supper Salad

2 medium potatoes
1 T. ea. minced parsley and green onion
1 T. salad oil, cold-pressed, sesame or olive
½ T. apple cider vinegar
Kelp and vegetable seasoning
⅙ c. eggless mayonnaise
¼ red onion separated in rings, thinly sliced
¼ bunch watercress, rinsed, drained and chopped
2 c. shredded salad greens, escarole, chicory and lettuce

1 large tomato cut in wedges
½ avocado sliced
½ cucumber cut in spears
½ bell pepper, seeded, sliced in rings
½ bunch radishes, cleaned

Slice potatoes, toss with parsley, green onion, oil, vinegar, kelp and vegetable seasoning. Add eggless mayonnaise or lecithinnaise from health food store. Chill until ready to serve. Arrange bed of watercress and greens on platter. Mound potatoes in center and arrange tomato wedges, avocado, cucumber, bell pepper and onion on greens surrounding potato salad. Have a side dish of sunflower seeds and pumpkin seeds. Have herb dressing available.

Rejuvenation Salad

4 large tomatoes, cubed
2 cucumbers, diced
2 stalks celery, diced
½ c. finely chopped onion, red
½ bunch watercress, chopped
¼ c. chopped parsley
Pinch of basil

Dried mint or 1 t. fresh mint
¼ c. lemon juice
2 T. cold-pressed oil
2 t. vegetable seasoning
Ground kelp to taste
Vegasal to taste

Combine tomatoes, cucumbers, celery, onion, watercress, parsley, basil and mint, then toss. Sprinkle with lemon juice, oil, vegetable seasoning and kelp. Then toss again. You may omit oil.

Golden Cole Slaw

1 c. shredded carrots
1 c. shredded rutabaga

1 c. shredded cabbage
Unsweetened shredded coconut

Toss the shredded vegetables together lightly with just enough salad dressing to moisten. Sprinkle with coconut. These vegetables make a delightful flavor combination.

Cole Slaw

6 c. shredded cabbage
½ c. coarsely chopped salted nuts

Combine and add enough salad dressing to moisten.

Chinese Salad Fit for a Mandarin

4 baked chicken breasts shredded
1 pkg. Chinese vermicelli noodles
Chinese spice
Cinnamon salt
1 t. cottonseed oil

½ c. sesame seeds
1 bunch Chinese parsley
Cilantro (tough to find
 but worth the trouble)

Saute shredded chicken in cottonseed oil and sesame seeds. Mix sauted chicken with all other ingredients, seasoning with spice and cinnamon salt. This one is worth the extra trouble — it's the best Chinese salad you will ever taste.

Chop Suey Salad

Cabbage
Parsley
Bok Choy

Watercress
Green onions
Lettuce

Raisins

Finely shred cabbage and mix well with parsley, bok choy, sprigs of watercress and young green onions. Arrange on a bed of lettuce and pour tofu dressing over the top. Sprinkle with raisins and nuts and apricot kernels.

SALAD DRESSINGS

Herb Dressing

¼ t. thyme, ground
¼ t. marjoram, ground
¼ t. tarragon, ground
½ t. basil, ground

½ c. cold pressed oil
3 T. apple cider vinegar
1 T. finely chopped fresh parsley
1 t. sea salt or 1 t. kelp

Shake vigorously in covered jar until blended. Allow to stand in refrigerator until flavors are blended.

Lemon Herb Dressing

Celery seed to taste
1 green onion with tops,
 chopped very fine
1 t. vegetable broth & seasoning
½ t. sea salt or kelp

2 sprigs parsley
¼ t. dried sweet basil
⅔ c. cold-pressed salad oil
1/16 t. marjoram
Juice of one lemon

Shake vigorously and cover jar until blended. Allow to stand in refrigerator until flavors are blended.

Garlic Herb Dressing

Use the same basic recipe as in lemon herb dressing eliminating the lemon juice. Add ⅔ cup apple cider vinegar, ¼ t. dry mustard and 1 clove garlic peeled and split. After the flavors are blended the garlic may be discarded a day or two later.

Cucumber Salad Dressing

1 c. eggless mayonnaise	½ c. cucumber
Pinch of dill	Season to taste

Golden Salad Dressing

1 c. water
¼ c. flour, unbleached or whole
   wheat pastry or millet flour

Blend well and remove from blender to sauce pan. Boil 5 minutes stirring constantly. Cool and return to blender. Add ½ cup raw carrots cut in pieces, ½ t. salt, 1 T. honey, 1 clove garlic or 1 T. chopped onion, ½ cup water, 1 T. lemon juice. Blend until smooth; refrigerate.

Variations: For fruit salad use apple in place of carrot and omit onion and garlic.

Taste Tempting Dressing

To 1 quart eggless mayonnaise from the health food store, add:

¼ c. chopped parsley	¾ t. oregano
¼ c. chopped green peppers	⅛ t. garlic powder
2 t. sweet basil	⅛ c. lemon juice
1½ t. dill weed	⅛ c. plus tomato sauce
½ t. thyme	¾ t. Maggi
½ t. marjoram	¾ t. salt

Stir gently until all is well mixed.

Thousand Island Dressing

2 c. mayonnaise

1 T. green pepper chopped fine

1 T. onion chopped fine

1 T. pimento

2 T. tomato sauce

¼ t. dill weed

4 to 6 ripe olives diced fine

Stir together until well mixed.

Low Calorie French Dressing
(for the diet conscious)

1 c. tomato juice

½ c. grapefruit juice

½ c. vegetable boullion (½ t. chicken-like seasoning or vegetable seasoning with ½ cup water)

Mix together well. Yield 2 cups.

Cole Slaw Dressing

½ c. mayonnaise

1 T. honey

1 t. lemon juice

½ t. celery seed

½ t. onion salt

Mix all together well.

Fruit Salad Dressing #1

1 c. orange juice

1 T. Tahini or 1 T. almond nut butter

1 t. honey

Stir together or blend in blender.

Golden Dressing for Fruit Salads

2 to 3 T. honey

1½ T. cornstarch

½ c. pineapple juice

1 T. grated orange peel (organic)

2 T. lemon juice

2 T. orange juice

Mix honey and cornstarch in sauce pan. Stir in pineapple juice and cook until thick, stirring constantly. Add and blend in rest of ingredients. Cool. Yield 1 cup.

Avocado Salad Dressing

1 large ripe avocado
1 T. lemon juice
1 T. minced onion
2 T. chopped pimento or
  red bell pepper
½ t. salt
2 T. mayonnaise

Mash avocado with fork. Add rest of the ingredients. This is in the fourth day lunch menu.

Mushroom Salad

⅓ c. clam juice
⅓ c. oil
2 T. vinegar
½ t. sea salt
¼ t. tarragon
¼ lb. mushrooms, sliced
1 red onion, thinly sliced
1 to 1½ qt. salad greens —
  Escarole, chicory, Boston and
  leaf lettuce, crisped
1 tomato cut in wedges

In a glass or ceramic bowl, combine the clam juice, vinegar, salt and tarragon. Beat with a rotary beater until well blended. Add mushrooms and onions and chill well. Place crisp salad greens (spinach if desired) in a salad bowl. Add mushroom-onion mixture and toss. Garnish with tomato wedges and serve immediately.

Zucchini Salad

3 small young zucchini,
  about 1 lb.
3 scallions finely chopped
2 T. snipped fresh dill weed
1 T. chopped parsley
¼ t. oregano
1 cup yogurt
1 T. lemon juice
1 t. honey

Wash zucchini and dice very fine. Place in a salad bowl with scallions, dill, parsley and oregano. Combine the yogurt, lemon juice and honey and pour over the zucchini and toss to mix well. Refrigerate 30 minutes or longer before serving.

Raw Beet Salad

1 bunch small young beets, tops
  removed for a tossed salad bowl
¼ c. honey
¼ c. oil

2 c. shredded red cabbage   Sea salt, Vegasal or Spike to taste
1 c. shredded carrots
½ c. lemon juice

Grate the beets finely into a salad bowl. Add the cabbage and carrots. Mix together lemon juice, honey, oil and salt and pour over beet mixture. Toss and chill well.

Apple Slaw

1 small head green cabbage,   1 T. chopped green pepper
  finely shredded   1 large apple, cored and finely
1 carrot grated   chopped
2 T. chopped celery   1 T. grated onion

Dressing:

1 T. honey   1 T. vinegar
½ t. sea salt   1 T. eggless mayonnaise
few grains cayenne pepper

Combine cabbage, carrot, celery, green pepper, apple and onion in a salad bowl. Beat together the dressing ingredients. Pour over the salad and toss well. Let stand at least 20 minutes in refrigerator before serving.

Caesar Salad Dressing

¼ c. lemon juice   1 clove garlic finely chopped
¼ c. water   1 T. anchovy paste
¼ c. cider vinegar   1 T. honey
¼ to ½ t. vegetable salt   3 T. grated Romano cheese
¼ t. fresh cayenne pepper   ¾ c. cold pressed oil

Put all ingredients except oil in blender. Blend until smooth. While blending add the oil gradually on medium speed until the mixture thickens. Chill well.

Russian Salad Dressing

1 c. cottage cheese (low fat)   ¼ c. tomato juice, approx.
1 T. vinegar or lemon juice   1 hard boiled egg, chopped

Put the cottage cheese, vinegar or lemon juice in electric blender. Add ¼ cup tomato juice and blend until very smooth, adding more tomato juice if necessary. Stir the egg into the dressing just before serving. Yields about 1 cup.

Apple Banana Salad

3 lbs. sweet apples, some red
and some yellow
2 or 3 bananas

1 c. macadamia nuts
Eggless mayonnaise
Boston lettuce cups

Core the apples but do not peel. Cut into bite size pieces and place in a salad bowl. Slice bananas and add to apple. Sprinkle with the nuts and toss with mayonnaise or with whipped nut cream. Serve in lettuce cups. About 6 servings.

California Fruit Salad

1 large cantaloupe cubed or made into melon balls
8 bananas, sliced
½ lb. fresh cherries, halved and pitted
1 pt. strawberries, halved
4 fresh peaches, pitted and sliced
1 fresh pineapple, peeled, cored and cubed
2 c. seedless grapes
1 c. mandarin orange segments, optional
1 can 8-oz. papaya juice or nectar
1 qt. canned or bottled guava juice
1 cannister low fat cottage cheese sprinkled with wheat germ

Combine all ingredients except cottage cheese in a large salad bowl. For extra crispness, watermelon is good in melon balls when in season. Chill for at least 3 hours. With an ice cream scoop, serve scoops of cottage cheese sprinkled with wheat germ with a lovely red strawberry on top.

Ambrosia Dressing
for California Fruit Salad

One cup mayonnaise with ½ cup raw, skimmed milk. Add 1 T. vanilla and 2 T. honey or to taste. Blend in blender. Add a pinch of nutmeg to taste.

Judy's Waldorf Cabbage Salad

¼ head fresh cabbage, grated or shredded
4 oz. fresh mushrooms, sliced
1 small onion, sliced
1 tart apple, cored and sliced
⅛ c. wheat sprouts
¼ c. alfalfa sprouts
¼ c. walnuts or cashews chopped
1¼ c. mayonnaise mixed with Honegar
Salt, pepper and kelp to taste

Place in serving dish and top with fresh tarragon and paprika.

Taiwan Fruit Salad

6 medium carrots, grated
1 pineapple, cubed (shell out pineapple) or 1 can pineapple
1 cup raisins
6 medium apples, cubed
⅔ c. raw macadamia nuts or raw cashews
1 cup coconut

Mix together and serve in cut pineapple shells.

American Fruit Salad

Cut into chunks:

1 pineapple	2 oranges
2 apples	3 bananas

Add macadamia nuts and cashews.

These ingredients are available all over America year-round. Suggested dressing for this is Judy's Blender Mix.

Judy's Blender Mix

½ c. raw wheat germ	¼ c. honey (or to taste)
2 c. plain yogurt	2 bananas
½ c. mayonnaise (optional)	1 t. cinnamon

California Fresh Fruit Salad

Cut into bite sizes: watermelon, cantaloupe, honeydew melon, fresh peaches and seedless green grapes. Mix together and sprinkle lime, lemon or honey over it or serve with Ambrosia Dressing or the whipped cream that is in the Back to Basics section.

Cole Slaw Rich in B-17

2 c. finely shredded cabbage
½ green pepper, diced
½ carrot, shredded
½ peeled cucumber, seeded
  and chopped
1 sweet onion, finely sliced
1½ T. sorghum

2 T. red wine vinegar
1 T. cold water
1 T. white vinegar
1 T. oil
1 T. sea salt or kelp
1 clove garlic, finely chopped

Combine cabbage, pepper, carrot, cucumber and onion in ceramic or glass bowl. Mix together the remaining ingredients and pour over the vegetables. Allow to marinate in the refrigerator a few hours or overnight. Serves 6.

Cashew Dressed Slaw

1 small head green cabbage, finely
  shredded
1 c. fresh pineapple
1 c. cashews, ground in food
  grinder

¼ c. water
¼ c. honey
2 T. cider vinegar
Kelp or Vegasal to taste

Place cabbage and pineapple in a salad bowl. Mix cashews with water to make a stiff paste. Add honey, vinegar and kelp to taste. Pour over cabbage and pineapple and toss. Serve 6-8.

Watercress Corn Salad

1 bunch watercress chopped to bite size
Kernels scrapped from 4 cobs of corn
¼ c. vegetable baco-bits

Mix all together. Use parsley dressing.

Parsley Dressing

1 bunch parsley
2 cloves garlic
1½ c. sesame oil

1½ c. lemon juice
1 t. mustard
Norwegian kelp for seasoning

Put garlic, oil and mustard in blender. Add chopped parsley and lemon juice to taste. Whiz briefly.

Marinated Broccoli Salad

1 bunch broccoli, broken into
   small flowerets
Boiling salted water
½ c. oil
½ c. lemon juice

Kelp or sea salt
Cayenne pepper to taste
1 clove garlic chopped

Put broccoli in a skillet with small amount of water. Steam the broccoli, cover and simmer until broccoli is crisp-tender. Meanwhile, beat together remaining ingredients. Pour dressing over broccoli. Chill well before serving.

Use stems from broccoli in following salad.

Grated Salad

3 c. grated cabbage
2 c. grated carrots
½ c. broccoli stalks
   (finely chopped)
⅓ c. sesame seeds ground
   or whole
1 tomato diced

½ avocado, peeled, pitted and
   cubed and dipped in lemon juice
   to prevent darkening
½ c. chopped cucumber
¼ c. chopped green pepper
¼ c. chopped celery

In a large bowl combine cabbage, carrots, broccoli and sesame seeds. Use the tomato, avocado, cucumber, green pepper and celery to garnish the salad in an attractive pattern. At the table toss with the dressing.

Herb Dressing

¼ c. apple cider vinegar
2 T. water
2 T. vegetable broth flavoring
   (Mr. Bronner's or Bi-Gor-Cup)
1 t. Meadowbrook brand salad
   herbs or your own choice of
   several herbs

1 t. sea salt or kelp
⅔ c. sesame oil

Put all ingredients except oil in a jar. Shake well. Add oil and shake again. Chill several hours before using.

Sesame Salad Dressing

½ c. ground sesame seeds
1 c. water, approx. (use water
   from steaming broccoli)

1 t. kelp
Juice of ½ lemon
½ clove garlic

Place seeds and 1 cup water in blender and blend until smooth. Add remaining ingredients and blend until smooth, adding more water if necessary to give correct consistency. Yield about 1 cup.

Note: Add ½ cup chopped onions, ½ cup chopped celery, and ½ cup mixed alfalfa, mung bean and lentil sprouts. Blend until smooth for a mock tuna sandwich spread.

Date Spread

1 cup chopped pitted dates   1 cup water

Cook together, stirring often to prevent sticking until dates are very soft. Whiz in blender briefly. Refrigerate. Keeps well one week.

Apple Date Spread

2 chopped apples
½ cup date spread

Whiz in blender until smooth.

Fruit Spread

1 ea. orange, yellow apple, banana

Blend together until smooth. Refrigerate. Will keep well one or two days.

Berry Sauce

For waffles, pancakes and as a topping on yogurt sundaes.

4 c. frozen, unsweetened berries, thawed
2 T. tapioca, ground
Juice and water to make 1½ cups liquid
1 to 2 very ripe bananas

Pour juice off berries into 2 cup measure. Add water to make 1½ cups and put in blender. Add bananas and tapioca. Whiz briefly.

Place in sauce pan and cook over medium heat until thickened. Add berries and heat through.

Pineapple and Banana Spread

¼ of a fresh pineapple, in chunks
2 bananas

Blend until smooth. Refrigerate. Will keep well for about 2 days.

Orange Spread

2 oranges
½ c. dried apricots or
4 fresh apricots

Whiz in blender until smooth. Refrigerate. Keeps well 2 or 3 days.

Applesauce

Whiz until smooth: 6 quartered, cored, unpeeled yellow apples. Include the apple seeds. With enough pineapple juice, approximately ½ to ¾ cup to blend, blend until smooth. Add date spread to sweeten, if desired.

Apricot Sauce

2 c. dried apricots   2 oranges
2 c. water   ¾ c. unsweetened pineapple juice

Soak apricots in water overnight. Put apricots, water and oranges in which they were soaked in blender. Whiz briefly. Add pineapple juice slowly while blending. Delicious on hot cereal, waffles, french toast, etc.

BACK TO BASICS

Cashew Milk

Into 2 qt. bottles measure 1½ cups cold water and set aside. Into the blender measure 1½ cups cashews. Add 1½ cups cold water, 2 T. honey, 2 t. vanilla, pinch of salt. Blend until smooth. Add 1 cup cold water and blend a few more seconds. Pour contents equally into each quart bottle. Rinse out blender with one cup water and pour that into bottles. Finish filling bottles with water from tap. Refrigerate immediately. (Strain if too grainy). Keeps a week or longer. May use sunflower seeds or sesame seeds.

Almond Fruit Milk

4 c. water
1½ c. almonds

⅛ t. salt
½ c. dried bananas, apples or
    fresh fruit

Grind almonds fine. Soak dried fruit in a cup of hot water 5 to 10 minutes to soften. Blend all ingredients until smooth. Use as cream on cereal.

Cashew Cream

1 c. water
½ c. cashews of almonds, blanched
1 t. honey, or 6 to 8 dates

Liquefy all together for 2 to 3 minutes. Delicious over cereal, etc. Be sure to wash raw cashews before using them.

Low Calorie Eggless Mayonnaise

Blend in blender 4 cups water, 1 cup millet flour. Put in sauce pan and cook until thick and bubbly. Stir constantly. Cool. Put 2 cups of the above into blender and add: 2 T. honey, 1½ t. salt, ½ t. garlic powder, ½ t. onion powder. Blend all of this, then slowly add: ½ to ¾ cup oil (until white and shiny); then add 2 T. lemon juice.

Home Style Mustard

1 cup mayonnaise
1 t. tumeric
2 t. onion juice (grate onion on fine grater or scrape with a paring knife)
2 T. chopped parsley
1 T. lemon juice
Dash of paprika, garlic and onion salt.

Mix all ingredients in a small bowl.

Quick Tomato Catsup

½ c. chopped onion	1 t. salt
1 minced clove garlic	1 t. paprika
¼ c. lemon juice	¼ t. cumin
2 c. tomato puree	½ t. sweet basil
1 c. tomato paste	¼ cup water

Blend onion and garlic with lemon juice and ½ cup tomato puree until smooth. Combine with rest of ingredients. Bring to a boil and let simmer a few minutes or until desired consistency. Makes 1 quart.

Lemon Juice Catsup

1 can tomatoes, 28-oz.	1 clove garlic, minced
½ can plain tomato paste, 6 oz.	½ pimento, diced
1½ t. salt	1 bay leaf
1 t. Savorex	½ t. basil
1 medium onion, chopped	¼ c. lemon juice
1 large stalk celery, diced	2 T. honey
2 sprigs parsley, chopped	

Simmer first 4 ingredients in heavy sauce pan while preparing vegetables. Add vegetables and all except lemon juice and honey. Simmer until vegetables are crispy tender. Remove bay leaf. This makes a tomato relish. For catsup, whiz in blender or press through sieve. Cool. Add lemon juice and honey. Refrigerate. This may be canned.

Energy Spread
(or eggless hollandaise)

This is in the 7th day lunch menu and 6th day dinner menu and is delicious.

1 c. mayonnaise	2 T. brewers yeast
½ t. turmeric	¼ t. soy sauce

Mix, chill and let stand 2 hours before serving on toast, bread or baked potatoes.

Tofu Cottage Cheese

½ cup tofu
¼ t. celery salt
⅛ t. onion powder or
1 t. chopped green onions

Pinch of garlic salt
¼ t. soy sauce

Mix together with fork to medium curd. 1 serving.

Soy Spread

⅓ c. soy flour
⅓ c. millet flour

Dextrinize on low heat at 300 degrees. Let cool. Mix with 1¾ cups water. Cook gently, stirring constantly, about 3 minutes. Reduce heat to a simmer and cook 10 minutes. Add ½ t. salt, 2 T. lemon juice, ¼ t. garlic powder, 1 t. honey. Stir well. Refrigerate. Keeps up to 2 weeks. Whip with a fork before serving. (May need to add water if it is too thick). Can be used as sandwich spread or mayonnaise.

Mushroom Gravy

4 T. flour mixed with enough water to make a smooth paste
2 T. minced onion
½ c. mushrooms
2 cups hot water (or 2 cups chicken stock)
¼ t. soy sauce
¼ t. Savorex
¼ t. salt

Combine onions and mushrooms in small sauce pan over low heat. Add small amount of water, if necessary, and cook until limp. Stir in flour mixture, add hot water and cook until slightly thickened. Add seasonings.

For thick gravy, 3 T. per cup of liquid. Makes approximately 2 cans of cream of mushroom soup.

Basic Tomato Sauce

12 large ripe tomatoes,
  skinned and chopped

2 T. snipped fresh chives
2 T. chopped parsley

2 green peppers, seeded	2 T. chopped fresh basil
2 onions, chopped	2 cloves garlic, chopped fine
2 carrots, chopped	Salt & pepper to taste
6 stalks celery, diced	½ t. Worcestershire sauce

Combine all ingredients in a stainless steel or porcelain steel pan or casserole. Bring to a boil and simmer uncovered for 45 minutes. Puree in a blender if desired.

Refrigerate overnight before using or freezing for future use. Yield about 2 quarts.

Barbecue Sauce

To ½ cup tomato sauce add juice of one lemon wedge, 1 clove garlic crushed, ¼ t. rosemary, ¼ t. sweet basil, a dash of honegar. Mix well.

Basic Millet Preparation

1 cup of water to 3 cups of millet. Place together in a covered pot on low heat. You may find a double boiler works better in the preparation of millet; cooking time 40 to 45 minutes. Remember to simmer this. Brown rice is cooked in the same method.

CHAPTER 16:

Breakfast Dishes

Millet Breakfast Cereal

1 c. whole hulled millet	1 c. chopped, unpeeled, cored apples
1 qt. water	1 c. raisins
1 t. salt	Sesame seeds (optional)

Put millet, water and salt in sauce pan. Bring to a boil, at low heat cover and simmer 45 minutes or until soft. Add apples, raisins, and sesame seeds. Add honey to sweeten, if desired. Serve with raw skimmed milk or omit apples and raisins and serve with hot fruit sauce. Serves 4 to 6.

Three whole grain cereals all to be cooked the same:

Cereal #1

½ c. millet	3 c. water
½ c. buckwheat groats*	1 t. salt
¼ c. barley	

Cereal #2

½ c. whole wheat	3 c. water
½ c. millet	1 t. salt
¼ c. whole rye	

Cereal #3

½ c. buckwheat groats*	5 c. water
½ c. brown rice	1 t. salt
¼ c. whole wheat	

---

*Buckwheat groats absorb more water than other cereal. One cup of groats to five cups of water.

Remember to use bottled water with all of these recipes as fluoridation is antagonistic to enzymes.

Cook ingredients from one of the above groups in an electric bean pot all night or steam on lowest heat of burner on range at night. Breakfast is ready when you get up. Serve with raisins, dates, nuts, etc. or with hot fruit sauce. Use other combinations of grains but keep selections to two or three grains.

Note: Of utmost importance is the change to low heat and very slow cooking after the grain is first brought to a boil. The slow cooking tenderizes the fiber without destroying enzymes, Vitamin B-17, minerals or other needed values. Whole grains may be cooked in a bean pot which is heavy enough to retain the heat and continue the cooking slowly. In short, maintenance of low temperatures is a paramount rule in cooking grains. Natural grains are an excellent source of B-17, B-1 and E. These are destroyed by high temperatures. Therefore, special attention should be given to the preparation of hot breakfast cereal.

Ground Whole Grain Cereal

Put whole kernels of wheat, barley, rye, soy beans, corn, millet in blender and blend at high speed until it is as fine as you wish. (Use a combination of three grains).

> 1 c. grains
> 2 c. cold water
> 1 t. salt
> Raisins, dates, other dried fruits (optional)

Cook in sauce pan, double boiler or steamer. Boil 5 minutes, cover tightly and turn off heat. Let stand, without removing cover, for 20 minutes. Wheat germ may be added to cereal before serving. Serve with raw skimmed milk.

Whole Grain Cereal — Thermos Method

In the morning put one cup of millet, whole or cut, to soak. In the evening add enough water to equal 3 cups. Bring to a boil with grain and salt. Pour into preheated thermos. Screw on cap and turn on its side until breakfast time the next morning. Serve as usual with raisins, dates or fruit sauce or with raw skimmed milk.

Note: Save leftover cereal and mix with legumes and seeds or nuts and seasonings for tasty entrees. Mix while breakfast cereal is still warm. Pack into loaf pan or make into patties and bake.

Breakfast Beans

Pick from any one of the wide variety of B-17 rich beans.

2 c. beans of your choice	1 large onion, chopped
6 c. boiling water	Pinch of basil, optional
2 t. salt	Slices of whole wheat bread

Sort and wash beans. Add to boiling water and bring back to boiling point. Turn off heat and let stand for one hour, covered. Bring to boil and simmer until nearly done. Add salt and finish cooking. Saute onion on low heat in own juice. Add a little water if necessary. Add to beans with enough water to make a soupy consistency. Simmer until beans are very tender. Serve on toast.

El Rancho Breakfast Limas

Why not for breakfast:

2 c. cooked lima beans	1 t. marjoram
1½ c. grated chedder cheese (white)	¼ t. celery seed
1 T. tamari soy sauce	2 T. nutritional yeast
1 c. tomato sauce	1 t. garlic powder
2 T. sesame oil, cold pressed	¼ t. cayenne powder
2 medium white onions, diced	Few sprigs watercress or Chinese
2 stalks celery, finely chopped	parsley
Juice of ½ lemon	

In a Chinese wok or large frying pan saute onion and celery in the oil until golden. Add tomato sauce, spices and yeast and stir well over a low heat. Add limas, grated cheese and continue to stir. Next add lemon juice and tamari sauce. Heat through and serve, adding remaining grated cheese to each portion. Top each serving with garnish of parsley and/or watercress finely chopped.

Triple Grain Cakes

¼ c. millet whole grain	¾ c. raw skimmed milk
¼ c. barley whole grain	1 t. salt
¼ c. oats whole grain	1 t. date spread

Soak grains overnight in ¾ cup cold water. Drain water from grains and place in blender with milk. Whiz 3 to 5 minutes. Add salt, date spread and blend another minute. Continue blending until fluffy and filled with air and cook immediately on a pan that has been lightly greased with lecithin oil or cold pressed sesame oil.

Griddle Cakes

2 c. soaked soy beans or	1 t. honey
2 raw potatoes	1 t. salt
1 c. water	2/3 c. whole wheat
1 c. raw skimmed milk	2/3 c. millet flour

Blend all ingredients except flour and place in bowl. Stir in flour. Spoon into medium hot griddle. Cover and let brown; turn and brown other side. Best if well cooked. Place on cookie sheet between paper towels in warm oven until served.

Millet Soy Waffles

2¼ c. water	½ t. salt
1¼ c. millet flour or 1 c. millet	1½ c. soaked soy beans (1 cup dry)
seeds	1 T. oil (optional)

Soak beans several hours or overnight in sufficient water to cover. Drain; discard water. Soaked, drained soy beans may be kept in refrigerator for a week or in freezer for longer periods. Keep on hand for immediate use.

Combine all ingredients until light and foamy, about ½ minute. Let stand while waffle iron is heating. The batter thickens on standing. Blend briefly. Pour into pitcher for convenience. Bake in hot iron for 8 minutes or until brown. Set timer for 8 minutes and do not open until time is up. Cook few seconds longer if iron sticks. Another trick here is to line the waffle iron with sesame seeds. The oil from the sesame seeds will oil the pan and keep the waffles from sticking. Of course, you will now have sesame seeds covering your waffles which isn't a bad idea. When serving a large number, bake waffles ahead. Cool, stack and cover with wax paper. Just before serving reheat in hot waffle iron, oven or toaster.

Cashew Oat Waffles

2½ c. water	1/3 c. raw cashews
1¾ c. old fashioned oats	½ t. salt

Blend all ingredients until smooth. Bake in preheated medium hot waffle iron 10 to 12 minutes. Do not open before time is up.

Eggless French Toast

¾ c. water	2 to 4 pitted dates
½ c. raw cashews	Pinch of salt

Whole wheat bread several days old or use toast (or millet bread toasted)

Whiz water, cashews and dates in blender. Dip bread in cashew mixture. Place on cookie sheet and under broiler to brown. Turn and brown on other side at 450° to 500°. Top with fruit sauce, sorghum, or sliced bananas.

Tahini French Toast

1 c. Tahini	½ t. salt
1½ c. water	Slices of whole wheat bread

Mix until smooth. Dip whole wheat bread into mixture — quick in, quick out. Let excess batter drip off. Brown on both sides in skillet.

Granola

Mix in a large bowl:

7 c. oats	1 c. millet flour
½ c. soy flour	1 c. coconut
¾ c. almonds, slivered	1 t. salt

Whiz in blender ¾ cup water, ¾ cup pitted dates, 1 T. vanilla. Add liquid to dry ingredients. Mix thoroughly. Put in large shallow pan and bake at 250°. Stir every 20 minutes to prevent burning and bake until golden brown and crisp, about 1½ to 2 hours.

Barley Millet Muffins

1 c. barley flour	½ c. dried apples, ground or
1 c. millet	1 cup fresh shredded apples
½ c. raisins	½ t. salt
¾ c. water	

Wash, quarter and core apples. Shred, cut side down, on medium shredder. Pack into cup. Combine ingredients. Let stand for a few minutes to absorb moisture. Mix together firmly with fingers or fork. Spoon into oiled muffin tins, or use ice cream scoop. Fill pans well and round nicely. (If fresh shredded apples are used, combine apple with water and oil and then add to dry ingredients.) Bake at 350° for 25 minutes.

Breakfast Cookies

3 bananas	½ t. salt
1 c. chopped dates	1 T. vanilla
½ c. chopped nuts	2 c. quick oats

Mash bananas leaving some chunks; add dates and nuts. Beat well and add salt, vanilla and oats. Drop from spoon onto ungreased cookie sheet. Bake 25 minutes or so in 400° oven. Loosen immediately. Some cookie sheets may need a little oil. The very, very shiny ones need the least. If you need a bit of oil, lightly cover the pan either with lecithin oil or cold pressed sesame seed oil.

CHAPTER 17:

Home Made Breads

Common Defects In Bread and Their Possible Causes from *The Art of Making Bread* by Marian Dakin

1. Sour taste — period of fermentation too long, or temperature too high while fermenting, causing formation of acid; poor yeast or stable yeast starter.

2. Dry or crumbly — too much flour in dough; overbaking.

3. Heaviness — unevenness of temperature while rising. Insufficient kneading.

4. Cracks in crust — cooling in a draft; baking before sufficiently light; oven too hot.

5. Too thick a crust — oven too slow, baked too long; excess of salt.

6. Dark patches or streaks — poor material; shortening added to liquid before flour, thus allowing flour particles to become coated with fat before they had absorbed equal amounts of liquid.

7. Sogginess — too much liquid; insufficient baking.

8. Ill-shaped loaf — not molded well originally; too large a loaf for the pan; fermentation period too long; failure to rise to greatest size in oven.

9. Coarse grain — too high a temperature; fermented too long; too long rising in pan; oven too cool at first; pan to large for size of loaf.

Basic Bread Recipe

1 c. rolled oats
2 c. boiling water
1 large apple
½ c. pitted dates
2 T. yeast or 2 pkgs. dried yeast
7 to 8 c. flour (5 c. whole wheat, 3 c. millet flour)
1½ t. salt

Put oats into a large bowl and pour on boiling water. Let sit until water is absorbed, about 20 to 25 minutes. Wash and cut up apple. Put into blender with the dates and enough warm water to equal 1½ cups liquid. Blend very well. Pour into a large bowl. Add the yeast and stir in. Let sit 10 minutes or until bubbly. Combine the salt with the flour. When yeast mixture is ready, and the special ingredients of the day (see variations below), stir in flour 2 cups at a time beginning and ending with rye and millet flour. Knead. Leave dough in bowl, scatter ½ cup flour on top of dough and with heel of hand press into the dough with one quick firm press. With the fingers, get hold of the dough and sift it around, sometimes turning it over. Repeat this process over and over with the rest of the flour. If dough is sticky, work in a little more flour. Shape dough into a mound in center of bowl and cover with damp towel. Let rise about 2 hours until double in bulk. Punch down. Divide and place into 2 lightly oiled bread pans, shaping dough out to ends to cover pans. Cover and let rise again until the top is well rounded — about 1 hour. Bake 50 - 60 minutes at 350° on rack about 4 inches from bottom of oven.

1 c. seedless raisins and ¾ c. citron dried, fruits & peels
2 t. leaf sage, crumbled
1 t. leaf marjoram
1 t. dried basil
½ t. dried parsley
2 t. dried summer savory
1 t. anise seed
½ t. caraway seed

These variations can be used singularly or in conjunction.

Orange Raisin Nut Bread

Use 2 cups near boiling orange juice instead of water. Add 1 t. grated orange rind, 1 cup seedless raisins, ½ cup chopped walnuts.

Dark Mixed Grain Bread

½ c. wheat germ
½ c. buckwheat flour
1½ c. rye
4½ c. whole wheat

Pumpernickel

1 T. caraway seeds added to oatmeal mixture
1 c. bran flakes
2½ c. rye
3½ c. whole wheat flour

CHAPTER 18:

Main Entrees

Eggplant Parmesan

1 large eggplant
6 large tomatoes, skinned
1 lb. non-pasteurized Mozzarella cheese, thinly sliced
Basil, thyme, Italian seasoning, oregano & paprika

Preheat oven to 400°. Peel the eggplant and slice crosswise into paper thin slices. Blend the tomatoes in blender until smooth. Butter a large casserole or baking dish and make alternating layers of eggplant, Mozzarella and tomato puree, making the top layer cheese. Bake 1 hr. Serves 6.

½ lb. of whole milk, unpasteurized Ricotta can be added in layers, and zucchini cut into lengthwise strips can be substituted for eggplant.

Tofu Pie Filling

1 medium onion
¾ c. mushrooms, sliced
1 medium size zucchini squash, sliced
1 pkg. Tofu
1 c. grated cheese, optional
1 T. Olive oil
1 T. tamari
1 t. kelp, Norwegian
½ t. cooking wine, optional
1 pinch basil, thyme
2 pinches coriander
1 light pinch cayenne pepper
1 t. sea salt

Saute onions in liquids and oil until translucent. Add mushrooms, zucchini, herbs and spices to mixture in pie shell. Blend Tofu to ¾ T. tamari until creamy. Add creamy mixture to pie. Bake at 350° for approximately 30 to 45 minutes. Add grated cheese to melt on pie after pie is removed from oven.

Tofu Pie Shell

½ c. buckwheat
½ c. millet
1/3 c. sesame seeds, ground, raw or toasted
1 T. sesame Tahini
2 T. tamari

Bring water to boil, adding grains. Drain, if there is water after cooking. Moisten grains with sesame Tahini and tamari. Mix with hands until dough is soft and place in greased pie plate.

Fritata

1 bunch spinach
1 bunch Swiss chard
4 zucchini
1 onion
1 clove garlic, minced
3 eggs
1 t. Italian herb seasoning
¼ c. whole grain bread crumbs, minced
½ c. parmesan cheese
Sea salt or kelp, and cayenne pepper to taste

Wash spinach, chard and zucchini. Drain. Steam swiss chard and spinach lightly and cool. Saute zucchini and onion in oil 5 minutes and cool. Mix cheese and bread crumbs, Italian seasoning into 3 eggs, add salt, pepper and mix with cooled vegetables. Vegetables can be left in refrigerator overnight. Grease pan and spread 2 t. sesame seeds in pan. Shake off excess seeds. Add all ingredients and put in oven at 300° for 25 minutes until firm.

Lentil Loaf
for the modified diet

2½ c. cooked lentils
1 c. cooked millet
1 egg, separated - beat white

1 large onion
1 T. parsley
1 t. leaf oregano

Blend all ingredients together with enough stock or bouillon made with vegetable seasonings to moisten. Add egg white. Turn into oiled loaf pan and bake at 350° for 50 to 60 minutes.

Sauce for Lentil Loaf

1 onion
2 T. arrowroot
2 c. cold water

1 T. safflower oil
2 T. vegetable seasoning
2 T. mushrooms

Saute mushrooms in 1 T. oil over low heat. Cover for 10 minutes. Remove from pan. In same pan saute chopped onion in 1 T. oil over low heat, covered, for 10 minutes. Add arrowroot and vegetable seasoning to 2 c. water. Mix well and add to onion. Return to pan and slowly bring to a boil. Turn down heat and simmer until thickened. Add mushrooms and serve over lentil loaf.

Vegetable Plate with Lima Beans and Green Beans

Place a large baked potato in center of dinner plate and surround it with baby lima beans, green beans, broccoli, Swiss chard, sliced beets, carrots.

This combination is complete in vitamins, minerals, chlorophyll and nitrilosides and is alkaline in its content.

Vegetable Chow Mein

1 c. sliced celery
1 c. sliced onion
1 c. broccoli stalks, peeled & sliced
1 c. Chinese cabbage or plain
  cabbage

1 c. sliced mushrooms
1 c. broccoli flowerets
½ c. celery root, sliced
Vegetable seasoning
1 c. bean sprouts

Steam vegetables with ½ c. water over low heat for 15 or 20 minutes. (Bring to boil first). To 1 c. warm water add 2 t. vegetable seasoning; pour over vegetables. Add sprouts. Mix arrowroot with a little cold water; add carefully to vegetables. Add 2 T. margarine; stir carefully. Serve over brown rice.

Bob's Burgers

3 c. cooked bulgar	½ t. garlic
10 mushrooms, sliced	2 T. tamari sauce
1 egg	1 T. tarragon
1 whole onion, chopped	3 T. Whole wheat flour
¼ c. green bell pepper, chopped	2 c. grated cheese

Mix all ingredients with the bulgar. Form into patties. It should make about 11 patties. Place under broiler for about 5 minutes or until tops are golden brown.

Meatless Spaghetti Sauce

½ c. lentils, cooked	1 t. onion powder
2 c. red kidney beans	1 t. garlic powder
2 c. tomatoes, chopped	1 t. chives
2 whole onions, chopped	1 t. parsley
½ t. sea salt	½ c. tomato juice
1 c. sliced mushrooms	2 T. olive oil
2 stalks celery with tops, chopped	Water, just as little as possible
2 T. oregano	so that spaghetti is thick.
¼ t. cayenne	

Boil a quart of water and drop in lentils and kidney beans with 2 bay leaves. Then turn off the heat. Allow the beans to sit one hour. Pour off the excess water and reserve it for later. Put in remaining ingredients and simmer. Add the water you reserved earlier, if needed. Pour over spaghetti noodles.

Curried Pea Soup

2 c. dried split peas	½ t. celery seed
10 c. water	½ t. curry powder
1 carrot, grated	2 c. cooked brown rice
2 potatoes, grated	½ c. grated apricot kernels.
1 onion, grated	

Place split peas in a large soup pot with 10 c. water. Bring to a boil, cover and cook over low heat about 1 hour. Meanwhile, grate the vegetables.

After peas have cooked about 1 hour, add the grated vegetables, the celery seed and curry powder. Cover and cook for 30 minutes. Add the cooked rice. Cook about 30 minutes more before serving. Serves 6.

Stove Top Stew

3 onions, sliced	1 stalk broccoli, sliced (optional)
4 cloves garlic, pressed	1 lg. can tomatoes, (28 oz.) chopped
4 potatoes, chunked	2 T. molasses
4 stalks celery, sliced	1 T. parsley flakes
4 carrots, sliced	2 t. dill weed
2 zucchini, chunked (optional)	¾ c. burgundy wine (optional)
½ lb. mushrooms, sliced (optional)	3 T. arrowroot

Put ½ c. water in a large pot, add onions, garlic, potatoes, celery and carrots. Saute about 15 minutes. Add optional broccoli if desired, along with burgundy wine. Cover and steam vegetables about 10 minutes. Add tomatoes, molasses, parsley, dill, and optional zucchini and mushrooms, if desired.

Cover and simmer over low heat about 30 minutes longer. Serves 8.

This may be made ahead and reheated just before serving. Other vegetables may be used in place of optional ones, or they may be omitted.

Spinach-Rice Casserole

1 onion, chopped	1 t. cumin
2 c. spinach, chopped	2 tomatoes, sliced
3 c. cooked brown rice	½ c. apricot kernels
1 T. tamari	

Saute onion in a small amount of water until translucent. Add spinach and steam (covered) until barely tender (about 5 minutes). Remove from heat. Mix the rice with the onions and spinach. Press into lightly oiled baking dish (9 inch square or 12″

x 7″). Layer sliced tomatoes over the top. Bake 30 minutes at 350°. Serves 6.

Helpful Hints: Try sage, oregano or basil. Serve with gravy, if desired.

Sweet and Sour Lentil Stew

1/3 c. raw brown rice	1 clove garlic, crushed
1 c. uncooked lentils	1 bay leaf
4 c. water	½ t. basil
1 onion, chopped or sliced	1 T. tamari
1 carrot, chopped or sliced	1 T. lemon juice
2 potatoes, chopped	1 T. molasses
1 green pepper, chopped	½ T. cider vinegar
1 c. fresh tomatoes, chopped	

Put lentils, rice and water in a large pot. Bring to a boil. Reduce heat, cover and simmer for 30 minutes. Add onions, carrots, potatoes and green pepper. Simmer for 30 minutes more. Add tomatoes and seasonings. Cook an additional 30 minutes. Serve hot. Serves 6.

Helpful Hints: One 16 oz. can of tomatoes may be used instead of the fresh tomatoes. Other vegetables may be added as desired. Longer cooking ones should be added with the onions. Shorter cooking ones may be added with the tomatoes.

Vegetables and Rice

3 c. cooked brown rice	1 c. mung bean sprouts
1 onion, chopped	1 c. alfalfa sprouts
1 carrot, sliced	¼ t. basil
1 c. broccoli, sliced	¼ t. paprika
1 c. cauliflower, sliced	¼ t. sage
1 c. mushrooms, sliced	¼ t. marjoram
2 zucchini, sliced or cubed	

Begin with onion, carrot, broccoli and cauliflower. Saute in a small amount of water (½ c.) until crisp-tender; or steam in steamer basket until crisp-tender (15-20 minutes). Then add mushrooms, zucchini and mung bean sprouts for another 10 minutes. Then add the cooked rice and alfalfa sprouts and spices.

Heat for about 5 minutes and serve. Serves 4, as a main dish.

Helpful Hints: Cook rice early in the day and refrigerate or cook a large amount on one day to use in several different recipes. Rice also can be frozen. Vegetables can be changed as desired. Begin with longer-cooking ones, then add short-cooking ones.

Lentil-Rice Burgers

1 c. dried lentils (2 cups cooked)
1 c. short grain brown rice, raw (2½-3 c. cooked)
1 onion, chopped
1 t. sage

Cook lentils and rice separately until done. Drain water off lentils and mash with potato masher. Saute the chopped onion in ¼ c. water about 10 minutes. Combine the mashed lentils, the rice, onion and sage. Moisten hands and form into patties. Place on ungreased baking sheet. Bake in a 325° oven for 30 minutes. Serves 8.

Helpful Hints: Serve with gravy or a tomato sauce. Try them on whole wheat bread, or in pita bread, with tomato, lettuce, sprouts, etc.

Sloppy Lentils

2 c. dried lentils
1 large chopped onion
1 carrot, chopped
1 green pepper, chopped
4 c. water
4 c. tomato sauce

1 T. parsley flakes
1 bay leaf
½ t. basil
¼ t. garlic powder
1 T. salt-reduced tamari

Place lentils, onions, carrots and green pepper in a large pot with 4 c. of water. Cover and simmer for 30 minutes. Add tomato sauce and seasonings to the pot and simmer for 30 minutes longer. Serve over whole grain bread or muffins or over whole grains. Serves 6.

Helpful Hints: May be made ahead and reheated. Also freezes well.

Herbed Green Beans

1 lb. fresh green beans
½ t. basil
½ t. marjoram
½ t. chervil

1 t. parsley flakes
1 t. chives
⅛ t. thyme
⅛ t. summer savory (optional)

Wash and trim beans. Cut into 2 inch pieces. Place in pot with steamer basket and about 2 cups water (under the steamer basket). Steam until crisp tender, about 20 minutes. Combine the herbs in a small bowl. When beans are done, drain off water, place in serving bowl. Add the herb mixture, toss beans lightly to coat with mixture. Serve at once. Serves 4.

Stuffed Pita Bread

1 pkg. whole wheat pita bread
2 c. refried beans or garbanzo puree
2 chopped tomatoes
1 bunch chopped green onions
1 - 2 c. alfalfa sprouts *or* shredded lettuce
1 chopped green pepper (optional)
1 chopped cucumber (optional)
1 grated carrot (optional)
½ c. Mexican style chili salsa (Ortega)

Heat the bean mixture over low heat until heated through. Place in serving bowl. Place chopped vegetables on table in individual bowls. Let everyone assemble their own pita.

Suggestion: Cut pita in half with scissors. Spread apart. Fill with some bean mixture. Then add garnishes as desired. Spoon a little hot sauce over the garnishes and enjoy. Serves 6 - 8.

Enchilada Sauce

¼ c. water
1 onion, chopped
3 cloves garlic, crushed
¼ c. chopped green chili
1 lg. (28 oz.) can tomatoes
½ t. basil

½ t. ground cumin
¼ t. ground oregano
1 c. water
1 T. tamari
3 T. arrowroot
¼ c. water

Place ¼ c. water, onion and garlic in a large saucepan. Saute about 10 minutes. Chop the tomatoes well, add them and the juice to the pan, along with the green chili and the spices. Simmer for 15 minutes. Mix the tamari in 1 cup water, add to the tomato mixture. Dissolve the arrowroot in ¼c. water, add to the tomato mixture stirring well. Simmer about 10 minutes longer over very low heat, stirring occasionally. Serve with vegetable or bean enchiladas, polenta, whole grains or pasta. Makes about 6 cups.

Helpful Hints: Bean enchiladas are great and easy to make. Buy a package of corn tortillas (frozen), make up a batch or refried beans, chop a bunch of green onions. Take 1 tortilla at a time, place it on the heated sauce, one side only. Remove carfully. On the saucy side, spread a line of refried beans, sprinkle on a few green onions, roll up tortilla and place in baking dish, seam side down. Repeat until all tortillas are used and lined up in baking dish. Pour the enchilada sauce over them. Bake at 350° for 30 minutes.

Vegetable Bean Soup

1 c. dried kidney beans	⅓ c. long grain brown rice or ½ c.
2 cloves garlic, pressed	broken whole wheat spaghetti
1 onion, chopped	2-3 tomatoes, cut in wedges
2 potatoes	¼ c. chopped parsley
1 carrot	¼ t. celery seed
2 zucchini	¼ t. marjoram
2 leeks	1 t. basil
¼ lb. cabbage (savoy is best)	1 t. oregano

Place beans in pot with 2 quarts water. Bring to boil, remove from heat and let rest 1 hour. Then add chopped onion, garlic and simmer for 1½ hours.

Chop potatoes in large chunks, do not peel. Slice carrots ½ inch and zucchini 1 inch thick, scrub; do not peel. Slice leeks and cut beans into 1 inch pieces. Add to soup pot along with seasonings. Simmer for 1 hour longer.

Thinly slice cabbage and add to soup along with rice or spaghetti. Simmer another 20 minutes. Add more water if too thick. Add tomato wedges the last 10 minutes, just before serving.

Helpful Hints: Kidney beans make a good rich broth, but any other bean may also be used. Soup freezes well so make a large batch when you have time and freeze half for use on a busy day. Try using some chopped spinach, instead of the cabbage. By changing the vegetables and beans used, the soup can be different each time you make it. A meal in itself. Serves 8 - 10.

Chinese Peas and Mushrooms

1 lb. Chinese peas, washed and ends trimmed
½ lb. mushrooms, sliced
½ T. tamari
¼ c. water

Saute the Chinese peas in the water and tamari for 10 minutes. Add sliced mushrooms. Cook an additional 5 minutes. Serve at once. Serves 4.

Helpful Hints: Peas and onion slices are also good. Try mushrooms and onion slices too.

Bean Mixtures

Preparation Time: 15 minutes
Cooking Time: regular: 3-4 hours
                slow-cooked: 8-10 hours

 # One

1 c. split peas
½ c. lima beans
½ c. white beans
   or garbanzos
2 t. basil
1 bay leaf
4 c. water

 # Two

1 c. kidney beans
½ c. pinto beans
½ c. white beans
½ t. chili powder
½ t. ground cumin
¼ t. oregano (ground)
4 c. water

REGULAR COOKING: Place all ingredients from either # One or # Two into a large pot. Bring to a boil. Reduce heat to low, cover, and cook 3-4 hours until tender. Stir occasionally and add more water if necessary.

SLOW COOKING: Add all ingredients from either # One or # Two to your slow cooker. Stir. Cover and cook for 8-10 hours on low. Will cook in about 5 hours on high. Times may vary slightly due to differences in slow cookers.

Helpful Hints: A chopped onion may be added to either of the above recipes. Also 1 clove of crushed garlic may be used. These mixtures freeze well — good for a fast meal later. Add some pure vegetable seasoning if desired. Great over toast, griddle cakes, rice, potatoes, etc.

***

CREPES

Basic Whole Wheat Crepe Recipe

3 eggs	1½ c. millet
1 c. soy milk or raw milk	1 T. wheat germ
1¼ c. water	Pinch of salt
½ c. whole wheat flour	2 T. butter, melted

Place all ingredients in a blender or mixer and beat well. It is necessary to occasionally stir the batter. Fill the whole wheat crepes with crumbled tofu or chicken curry, or chicken and bean sprouts, or fresh sprouts and mushrooms, (see recipes below) or garbanzo sandwich filling.

Main Entree Crepe Filling:

Chicken Curry

1 3-4 lb. chicken fryer, organic, cut up
1 onion
2 stalks celery
2 whole cloves
1 bay leaf
1 to 2 T. Savorex or Dr. Bronner's Chicken Seasoning
   (like chicken bouillon)
Sea salt and cayenne to taste
Spring water

In large kettle simmer above ingredients for about 1 hour or until chicken is tender. Reserve broth, strain. Remove chicken from bones and cube.

3 T. butter or soy margarine	1 to 3 T. curry powder
3 T. millet flour	Salt and pepper to taste
2 to 3 c. reserved chicken broth	

Melt butter in sauce pan; add flour and chicken broth. Cook slowly until desired thickness. Add cubed chicken and seasoning. Arrange folded cubes on platter. Let guests choose their own topping of the following condiments: raisins, finely chopped almonds or macadamia nuts mixed with crushed apricot kernels, chopped fresh onions, sprouts, chutney, chopped sweet pickles, scallions, minced fresh parsley. (Cancer cells do not grow in potassium and parsley has plenty of potassium).

Chicken Bean Sprout Crepes

1 can (10¾ oz.) Cream of Chicken soup, or see "Back to Basics" Guide
2 c. diced chicken
1 8-oz. can water chestnuts, sliced
¼ c. white wine or milk (nut, soy or raw)
Bean sprouts
Dash of salt, sea or kelp
Paprika
Cayenne
Worcestershire

Mix all ingredients together in saucepan and heat. Top with sliced nuts and apricot kernels.

Fresh Mushroom Sprout Crepes

4 T. butter	3 T. millet flour
2 c. bean sprouts	1 c. milk (raw, soy, nut)
2 c. fresh mushrooms, sliced	Cayenne pepper & salt to taste
3 green onions, chopped	½ c. soy cream, raw

Melt butter. Saute onions and mushrooms. Add flour and stir. Add milk gradually, cooking over low heat until thickened. Before serving stir in sour cream for flavor and top with fresh bean sprouts.

Variation: Place filled mushroom crepes in buttered casserole. Cover with cheese sauce. Grate about ½ c. additional cheese, or sprinkle with parmesan cheese. Heat in oven until bubbly. Serve.

An added luxury to your kitchen might be an electric crepe maker. They are not terribly expensive and make ordinary foods seem unusual and festive. I have to admit I have an electric crepe pan which makes perfect crepes every time but the same can be done with a flat skillet which distributes heat evenly.

CHAPTER 19:

Desserts

Basic Dessert Crepe

¾ c. whole wheat flour
¾ c. millet
2 T. honey
Pinch of salt
3 eggs

1½ c. raw milk (dry soy milk can
  be substituted)
2 T. butter, melted
½ t. lemon, rum or vanilla
  extract

Place all ingredients in blender or mixer and beat well. Let batter stand one hour for more perfect crepes. Place filling in middle and fold all sides in to make pocket or make roll. Fill dessert crepes with fresh stawberries and sour cream or apples.

Apple Filled Crepes

⅓ c. butter
3 lbs. tart cooking apples

½ c. honey
1 t. cinnamon

Melt butter over medium heat. Add apples and mix with honey and cinnamon. Cook, stirring gently from time to time, until apples have softened and begin to change color. Fill crepes and fold. Sprinkle with chopped apricot kernels. Serve hot.

Use your imagination. All kinds of fresh fruits and berries can be used fresh and whipped nut milk makes a delicious topping.

Crepes and Fruit Spread: Crepes served with hot fruit sauce, apricot, berry, apple, date, pineapple, banana, orange, applesauce are delicious. Top with whipped nut cream and chopped nuts or apricot kernels.

Carrot Cake

From one of the world's finest pastry cooks, Florencia Joyce.

2½ c. unbleached flour	1¾ c. honey or date sugar
5 t. baking powder	1 c. safflower oil
½ t. cinnamon	1 c. chopped walnuts
¼ t. orange peel	1 c. raisins
¼ t. lemon peel	1 c. water
3 egg whites	2 c. carrots

Grate carrots. Chop walnuts. Sprinkle raisins with flour. Sift flour and baking powder, add orange and lemon peel and cinnamon. In a large bowl beat honey and oil. In a small bowl beat egg whites until frothy — set aside. Add water to honey and oil mix. Add flour mixture and mix well. Add raisins, walnuts, grated carrots, mixing after each addition. Fold in egg whites. Place in a 9x13 glass baking dish. Sprinkle top with raw sugar and chopped walnuts. Place in 350° oven and bake for 40 to 45 minutes.

Note: when the modified diet permits, the whole egg may be used.

Carob Cake
(The best I have ever tasted!)

1 c. + 2 T. barley flour	½ c. carob
2½ t. baking powder	2 eggs or egg whites
1 t. vanilla	¾ c. honey
½ c. safflower oil	¾ c. water

Beat eggs, add honey. Beat. Mix carob, baking powder and flour. Add to mixture while adding oil and water alternately. Add vanilla. Bake at 350° for 35 minutes or until done.

Note: Egg whites are used on the strict diet.

Frosting

1 egg white
½ c. carob
½ c. honey

Beat egg white until stiff. While beating add honey. Add carob. Mix well. Frost cake in the usual manner.

Zucchini Cake

2½ c. whole wheat flour
2 c. zucchini squash, grated
1 c. slivered almonds
1 c. apricots, chopped
1 lime or lemon
1 c. safflower oil

1 c. honey
½ c. blackstrap molasses
2 eggs or egg whites
2 t. baking powder
1 c. water

Beat eggs. Add honey and molasses while beating. Grate rind of lime and add. Add lime juice. Mix flour and baking powder. Add flour, water and oil alternately. Add zucchini and apricots. Place in a 9x13 baking dish. Sprinkle top with slivered almonds. Bake in 350° oven for 40 to 45 minutes.

Apple Brown Betty

10 apples
½ c. date sugar
¼ c. safflower margarine, melted
½ c. chopped walnuts
½ t. cinnamon

12 slices coarse bread crumbs
½ c. raisins
Juice of 1 lime
½ c. apricot kernels

Peel and slice apples and sprinkle with lemon or lime juice. Place ½ c. bread crumbs in bottom of 9″ square baking dish. Sprinkle bread crumbs with cinnamon and a little date sugar. Dot with raisins and pour over a little melted margarine. Repeat twice more. Place a row of apples over the crumbs and sprinkle with a little cinnamon, date sugar and chopped walnuts. Add a little of the margarine, dripping it lightly over the apples. Cover and place in a 250° F. oven until apples are tender. Green apples take about 1 hour. Delicious apples take about 30 minutes. Dip honey over the top before serving.

Baklavá

4 c. apricot kernels (1 16-oz. pkg.) finely chopped
1 t. cinnamon
1 lb. filo or strudle leaves
1 c. butter or soy margarine, melted
1 12-oz. jar of honey

About 2½ hours before serving or up to two days ahead, grease 13x9" baking dish. In large bowl with spoon combine chopped apricot kernels and ground cinnamon until blended. Set mixture aside. In baking dish place 1 sheet of filo allowing it to extend up sides of dishes. Brush with some butter of margarine. Repeat to make five more layers of filo. Sprinkle with 1 cup apricot kernel mixture. Cut remaining filo into approximately 13x9" rectangles. Place one sheet of filo in baking dish over walnut mixture. Brush with butter or soy margarine. Repeat to make at least six layers, overlapping small strips of filo to make rectangles if necessary. Sprinkle 1 cup apricot kernel mixture evenly over filo. Repeat step 3, two more times, replacing filo on top of last apricot kernel layer. Trim any filo that extends over top of dish. With sharp knife cut all layers in a diamond pattern to make 28 servings. Bake in 300° F. oven 1 hour 25 minutes or until top is golden brown.

Meanwhile, in 1-qt. saucepan over medium low heat, heat honey until hot but not boiling. Spoon hot honey evenly over baklava. Cool in pan or wire rack at least one hour, then cover and leave at room temperature until serving time.

Carob Brownies

2 eggs	1 t. baking soda
¾ c. honey	¾ c. water
½ c. melted butter	⅓ c. carob, sifted
1 t. vanilla	1 c. whole wheat flour
1 banana	1 c. broken walnut pieces
½ t. sea salt	

Beat eggs slightly, add honey, cooled butter, vanilla and banana. Mix well. Then add the dry ingredients alternately with water. Add broken walnut pieces last. Butter and flour a 13x9" glass baking dish and bake exactly 23 minutes. Do not overbake. The oven should be set at 350°.

Carob Brownie Icing No. 1

⅓ c. honey	¼ c. sifted carob powder
¼ T. melted butter	4 T. water

1 c. non-instant dry powder milk   1 t. vanilla

Mix all the ingredients together. Use the milk as a dry powder. Beat until smooth. If more water is needed add 1 more tablespoon.

Carob Brownie Icing No. 2

4 T. melted butter   ⅓ c. honey
2 t. vanilla   ¼ c. sifted carob

Mix all the ingredients and beat until smooth. Can be placed on hot brownies. Also can be used as carob syrup.

Flourless Pie Shell

½ c. buckwheat   1 T. sesame Tahini
½ c. millet   2 T. tamari
⅓ c. sesame seeds, ground, raw
   or toasted

Bring water to boil adding grains. Drain if there is water after cooling. Moisten grains with sesame tahini and tamari. Mix with hands until dough is soft and place in greased pie pan.

Apple Filling

6 c. apples, thinly sliced   1 t. cinnamon
   peelings on or taken off   Dash nutmeg
1 whole apple, cored   1⅓ T. butter - lemon juice
½ c. honey

Place whole apple along with honey, cinnamon, nutmeg, butter and lemon juice into food processor or blender. Blend this to liquid. Arrange the 6 cups of sliced apples in unbaked pie crust and pour liquid mixture over apples. Place another pie crust or lattice work on top and cover with foil. Bake at 425° for 10 minutes and then 30 minutes at 350°. Uncover the last 10 minutes.

Mo's Avocado Pie

Pie Crust:

> 1 lb. dates, mashed
> ½ c. ground walnuts
> ¼ c. shredded coconut
> 4 T. coconut juice

Mix with your hands until mixture is a soft dough. Lightly grease pan with soy margarine. Cover pie plate.

Filling:

Mash 3 medium avocados. Add ½ c. crushed pineapple, 6 T. coconut juice, 4 to 6 T. pure maple syrup. Add 3 T. apple pectin to 3 T. heated pineapple juice. When juice thickens, add to filling and mix lightly. Fill in pie plate. To decorate, slice kiwi fruit.

Effervescent Champagne Punch
Non-Alcoholic and Zingy

> 4 qts. Calistoga water
> 2 large cans pineapple juice
> 2 large bottles grape juice
> ½ gal. apple juice
> 1 qt. red zinger tea

Steep red zinger tea into heavy concentrate and strain. Cool tea. Mix all ingredients together in 5-gal. container. Add Calistoga water to taste. Fill into cored pineapple and let strawberries or orange rings float on top with ice cubes.

A wondrous lady of my acquaintance, Carole Mehrtens, who is the most gracious hostess I know, takes the tofu pie shell (from this book) and mashes fresh papayas in it, topped with Macadamia nuts. An unforgettable treat from this memorable beauty.

Cancer Blocking Agents Found in Foods or, Foods Containing B17 Laetrile

Seeds
Alfalfa, sprouted/Chia
Flax, Sesame (unhulled)
Linseed

Vegetables
Wild Cabbage, Brussel sprouts
Brassica Oleoracea, Cauliflower
Broccoli, Turnip
Black mustard, White mustard
Radish, Kohlrabi
Shepherd's purse, Collard greens
Kale, Squash
Spinach, Sweet Potato
Watercress, Yams

Berries
Almost all edible wild berries contain vitamin B17 and in more abundance than cultivated berries.

Blackberries, Boysenberries
Chokeberries, Cranberry
Elderberry, Gooseberry
Huckleberry, Loganberry
Mulberry, Raspberry
Strawberry

Sprouts

Vitamin C content is 10 to 30 times richer when these sources are sprouted.

Alfalfa, Bamboo
Fava, Garbanzo
Mung/Wheat berries

Legumes

Chick peas, Garbanzos
Fava, Kidney
Lentils (sprouted), Limas
Mung (sprouted), Navy
Peas, Scarlet runners

Grains

Barley, Buckwheat groats
Chia, Millet
Flax, Oats
Rice (brown), Rye
Vetch, Wheat berries

All kernels and seeds of fruits except the citrus. Fruit kernels and seeds contain the highest concentration of B17 to be found in nature. So in cooking or eating any of these fruits, I try always to include the seed. Particularly delicious is the apricot kernel wrapped in a dried apricot, which detracts from the bitter taste of the kernel.

Fruits

Apple, Apricot
Cranapple (wild), Cherry (choke)
Currants, Nectarine
Peach, Pear
Plum, Prune
Papaya, Quince

Nuts

Bitter almonds are grown mostly in China and illegal in this country. Ordinary sweet almonds have no substantial B17 content.

Cashews, Macadamia

Miscellaneous

Sorghum molasses, Clover (white and red)
Wheat grass

APPENDIX II

Defenders of Unorthodoxy

"A free society has a great stake in protecting the unorthodox. It is through unorthodoxy that society grows. If unproven avenues are blocked what remains is already known and both progress and freedom are lost. Today's orthodoxy was yesterday's heresy and yesterday's orthodoxy is today's superstition. In today's quackery lies the emergence of future enlightenment. In the ultimate, the supression of the freedom of one individual creative mind will kill more people than all the government programs will ever save."
The National Health Federation Bulletin, *April 1980*

The National Health Federation was founded by Fred Hart and is the oldest health freedom organization in America. It has championed the cause of freedom of choice for 25 years. Its service comes from, and returns to health- and freedom-concious Americans and serves no vested economic interest. The principles embodied by the NHF have attracted outstanding leaders, among them, Betty Lee Morales, Dr. Kurt Donsbach, Kirkpatrick Dilling, Earl Irons, John Fink, Dorothy Hart, Paul Virgin, Don Picket and Andrew McNaughton.

Betty Lee Morales has long been a guiding force within the National Health Federation's executive board. She contacted Drs. E. T. Krebs, Sr. and Jr. in 1958 when she first began to hear from victims whose cancer was controlled with laetrile. It was her ability to take a complicated subject and translate it into simple terms that communicated the genius of the Krebs' cancer theory

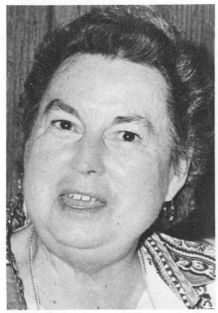

Betty Lee Morales

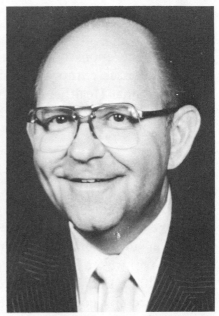

Dr. Kurt Donsbach

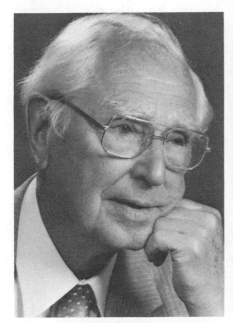

Earl Irons

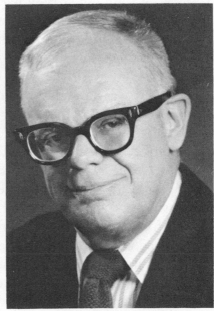

Kirkpatrick Dilling

to the American people. They welcomed an alternative to the state-sanctioned cut, burn, and poison techniques offered. Scion of three generations of preachers and naturopaths, Betty Lee holds audiences enraptured with the force of her message, at many National Health Federation conventions and civic affairs within this country and throughout the world.

Cecile Hoffman's last journey before her "impending" death was to be across the Pacific Ocean to Honolulu. It was spring of 1960. Her surgeon had given her six weeks to live. The purpose of Cecile's trip was to say goodbye to her mother. While awaiting their flight at Los Angeles International Airport her husband, Don, picked up a copy of Glen Kittler's book *Laetrile Control for Cancer*. They read of Andrew McNaughton's work with laetrile as head of the McNaughton Foundation, based in Montreal, Canada. Within hours they had changed both the direction and purpose of their flight and were on their way to Montreal.

From the fateful moment when Cecile and her husband read the Kittler book their thoughts changed from the death sentence she had received to the possible life-saving alternatives. For Cecile there was no such thing as false hope. Hope was hope in all its spirit-elevating reality.

Once in Montreal, they contacted Andrew. He referred them to a doctor in Montreal who was administering laetrile. Within two months, Cecile danced back into Andrew's office. The tumor had disappeared. In gratitude for her life, she asked Andrew, "What do I owe you?" Andrew replied, "You owe me a debt you will have difficulty in paying. What I ask in return is that you go out and spread the gospel of laetrile."

Cecile returned to the San Diego physician who had diagnosed her cancer as terminal. He refused to continue her laetrile shots or have anything whatsoever to do with her treatment. In desperation she found an obscure pathologist in Tijuana by the name of

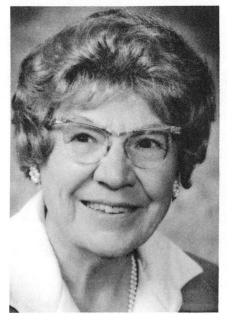

Dorothy Hart

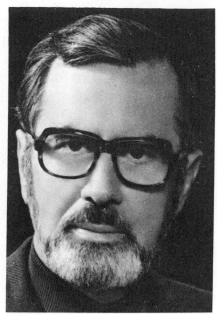

Andrew McNaughton

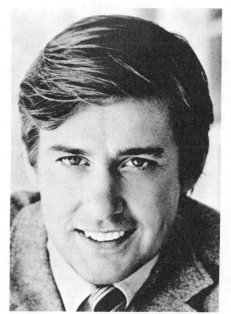

John Fink

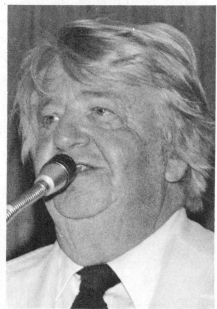

Ernst T. Krebs Jr.

Ernesto Contreras who had a small clinic named "The Good Samaritan". It all seemed so harmless to him to give this desperate woman the shots she felt had sustained her life.

Cecile's efforts to fulfill her debt to Andrew McNaughton to "go out and spread the gospel of laetrile," led her, in 1962, to establish the International Association of Cancer Victims and Friends. As a result of her treatment, she was pronounced free of cancer for almost 10 years. Cecile Hoffman lived those years educating other victims of cancer in the same life-giving alternative therapy that had extended her life for almost a decade. The work of the IACVF has since been carried through by Joe Koserik, Ms. Joe Czesny, and others.

In 1973 John Richardson, M.D., a physician in Albany, California, was arrested and sentenced to three years in federal prison for the crime of using a harmless fruit seed extract (laetrile) in the treatment of cancer. A group of 13 people gathered at that time to assist in his defense. One of them, Ed Griffin, christened the small group "The Committee For Freedom Of Choice". Under the guidance of these 13 men, committees began to spring up across the U.S. The committee at its onset served a useful purpose. All of the original founders except one have since resigned and disassociated themselves from the committee because of the rapacious motives that later dominated the committee.

In 1975 Judy Hall, the famous Country and Western singer from Alaska, was successfully treated for cancer at the Clinica Cydel, Mexico's finest alternative therapy clinic. Before leaving the border, she joint-drafted a bill with Andrew McNaughton to legalize laetrile in Alaska. On her return home, Judy gave the bill to Governor J. S. Hammond, whose wife was a cancer victim and later opted for laetrile treatment. Governor Hammond agreed to support the legislation. Thus, the first laetrile bill became law, setting the pattern for the 27 other states which, to this writing, have followed.

It was this historic event of 1975 which brought about a new era of political action to an idea whose time had come. In the face of massive political suppression, a handful of dedicated Americans began to motivate thousands more throughout the country and created a movement for freedom of choice unique in the history of our republic.

Betty Lee Morales, Cecile Hoffman and many other courageous Americans had planted the seeds that had finally begun to reap an effective harvest. This groundswell was now delivering some telling blows against the cancer establishment, expressing in action the ideals of many individual Americans.

In 1976, Glen Rutherford, a cancer patient, had had a tumor the size of a grapefruit on his colon. Under laetrile metabolic therapy it had disappeared in its entirety, as evidenced by X-ray. When Glen's supply of laetrile was confiscated, he threw down the gauntlet to the establishment with the resolve that "no government bureau is going to tell me how to die." On behalf of all dying cancer patients, he filed with attorney Ken Coe and later Kirkpatrick Dilling a class action suit against the FDA which filed in Federal Court, Judge Luther Bohanon presiding. In an eloquent statement for individual liberty, Judge Bohanon threw a restraining order against the FDA which allowed cancer patients to bring their medication in on a doctor-signed affidavit. In the December 5, 1977 decision, Judge Bohanon wrote:

"Having reviewed the decision of the Commissioner of Food and Drugs on Laetrile dated July 29, 1977 and the entire administrative record upon which that decision was based and the pleadings and briefs, the Court concludes that such decision is arbitrary, capricious, that it represents an abuse of discretion and is not in accordance with law. Consequently, it must be set aside and vacated. Individuals for whom no orthodox cure is available surely are entitled to select a health care approach with which they feel comfortable."

The issue appears largely unresolved as to laetrile's true effectiveness, in large part because the FDA has prevented adequate testing on humans.

While the Constitution does not explicitly mention a right of personal privacy, it is unchallengeable "that a right of personal privacy or a guarantee of certain areas or zones of privacy does exist under the Constitution.[1] This right has been discerned within the Bill of Rights and specifically within the language of the First, Fourth, Fifth, Ninth and Fourteenth Amendments to the Constitution... only personal rights that can be deemed fundamental or implicit in the concept of ordered liberty are included in this guarantee of personal privacy."

The freedom to care for one's health and person as coming within the purview of this right[2] comes under a right of privacy and has no more rightful place than in the physician/patient relationship.[3] The right to seek advice on one's health and the right to place reliance on the physician of one's choice are basic.

Judge Bohanon further commented:

"The right of privacy has been characterized more than once as simply the right 'to be left alone.' That right includes the privilege of an individual to plan his own affairs for outside areas of plainly harmful conduct; every American is left to shape his own life as he thinks best, do what he pleases, go where he pleases. Many knowledgeable and concerned individuals are questioning the effectiveness and wisdom of our orthodox approaches to combating cancer. The correctness of their criticism may not be determined for many years and, in any event, such discussion provokes controversies largely beyond the realm of the court's function.

"Nevertheless, it appears uncontrovertible that a patient has the right to refuse cancer treatment altogether; and, should he decide to forego conventional treatment, does he not possess a further right to enlist such nontoxic treatments, however unconventional, that he finds to be of comfort, particularly where recommended by his physician?

"Numerous cancer patients possess extensive firsthand experience with laetrile which has led them to believe, correctly or not, that the substance has eased their pain and

[1]Roe vs Wade, 420 U.S. 113, 152 1973.
[2]Doe vs Bolton, 410 U.S. 179, 213 1973.
[3]Doe, Supra at 219

prolonged their lives. Such personal convictions are not readily dispelled by government pronouncements or affidavits to the contrary. When deprived of treatment in this country, they go elsewhere and in so doing are denied close contact with their families and family doctors.

"Unintentionally, the FDA has brought needless hardship and expense to countless individuals required to travel to Mexico or Germany in order to utilize laetrile. If it were more readily available in this country, perhaps many patients currently obtaining the treatment abroad could be persuaded to remain under their doctor's care here and use the substance in conjunction with conventional treatments.

"Doubtless, FDA desires to protect the public. Such good intentions, however, are not the overriding issue. Many of us allocate time, money and other resources in ways susceptible to just criticism by many standards. Nonetheless, our political ideals emphasized that the right to decide is of much greater significance than the quality of those choices actually made. It is never easy for one who is concerned, and feels himself particularly knowledgeable, to observe others exercise their freedom in ways that appear to him unenlightened. As a nation, however, historically and continuously we are irrevocably committed to the principle that the individual must be given maximum latitude in determining his own personal destiny.

"To be insensitive to the very fundamental civil liberties at issue in this case and the fact that making the choice, regardless of its correctness, is the sole prerogative of the person whose body is being ravaged, is to display slight understanding of the essence of our free society and its constitutional underpinnings. This is notably true where, as here, there are no simple answers or obvious solutions, uncertainty is pervasive and even the best efforts leave so much to be desired."

With this federal judge's decision cancer patients could, for the first time, have access to their life-saving medication free from FDA persecution and prosecution.

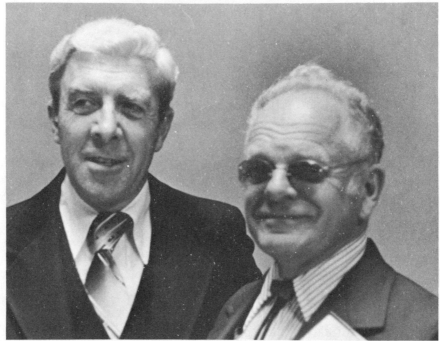

Dr. Harold Manner and cancer patient Glen Rutherford

The heat of political battle continued. As a result, many people became involved in this cause which they felt not only saved lives but preserved for themselves and generations to come their precious and hard-won freedoms.

Greg Kaye of New Jersey is an ardent and striving individual of exceptional dedication, eloquence and the kind of tenacity of purpose which typifies many of the defenders of nonorthodoxy. When he first met Dr. E. T. Krebs, Jr., the co-discoverer of laetrile, he offered any help he could render in the cause, but felt there was little he could do since he was not a bio-chemist, doctor or medical clinician. He did not understand Krebs' answer at the time: "You will soon realize that the medical problems of causation and treatment of cancer have been solved. Today cancer is a political issue." Over the years, Greg said, he has come to realize how right Dr. Krebs was.

After years of volunteer work, Greg spearheaded a New Jersey decriminalization bill in January 1978. This made laetrile metabolic therapy under the care of a physician a reality in New Jersey. The eastern sea coast state joined the roster of states which have, as of this writing, legalized the use of laetrile metabolic therapy.

In explaining laetrile metabolic therapy to the hundreds of patients who sit through the three-hour educational program Greg offers, he describes the therapy as "Laetrile being the hub of the modality, with many spokes supporting the wheel. Laetrile, along with vitamins, minerals and enzymes for immuno-support, diet and proper mental attitude, are all essential."

So important is mental attitude that it is ironic, says Greg, that patients always ask him who in his judgment, is the best physician

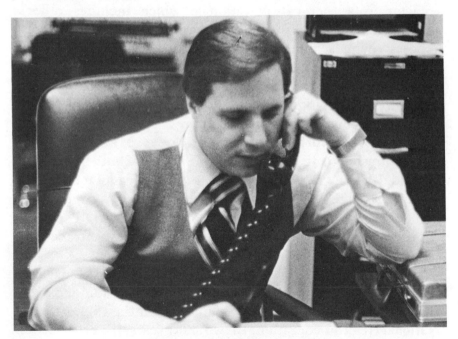

Greg Kaye of New Jersey

using laetrile. They are usually shocked by his answer that no such person exists. "I explain that the success I have seen over the years was brought by the knowledgeable patient who made a commitment to save his own life and that the physician's role is simply to supervise therapy." Patients must learn individual responsibility and positive mental attitude and we must stress this in the future.

Andrew McNaughton, recognized as a world leader in the struggle to legalize laetrile, concurs with Greg's opinion. McNaughton, the protege of E. T. Krebs, Jr., has worked to guide the orderly scientific development of laetrile with NCI and the FDA since the early 1960s. In a speech in San Ysidro in which Andrew was counseling a group of cancer patients from the Clinica Cydel, he said:

"These days we speak of the 'holistic approach to the metabolic therapy of cancer with vitamin B17.' Here laetrile is not regarded as a 'magic bullet' but rather as a central factor in a therapeutic rationale which includes other components such as nutrition; vitamin C in bowel-tolerance doses; vitamins, minerals and enzymes in proper physiological balance; enhancement of the immune system; appropriate rest and exercise; and, importantly, consideration of the mind/body relationship of each individual patient. Enlightened medicine today recognizes, as did the ancient peoples of the world, that total health involves a state of ease as contrasted to dis-ease in the functioning of both body and mind. Dysfunctions of the mind react with areas of metabolic weakness in the body, producing local conditions conducive to disease. In the words of Thornton Wilder: 'Despair probed the organs one by one, seeking the easiest entrance to the kill.'"

In November, 1978, *Public Scrutiny*, a monthly news magazine dedicated to the concept of freedom of choice, was founded by the author of this book, Maureen Salaman, with the support of the National Health Federation. In two short years, the pro-freedom forces, anxious for a publication with no financial vested interest,

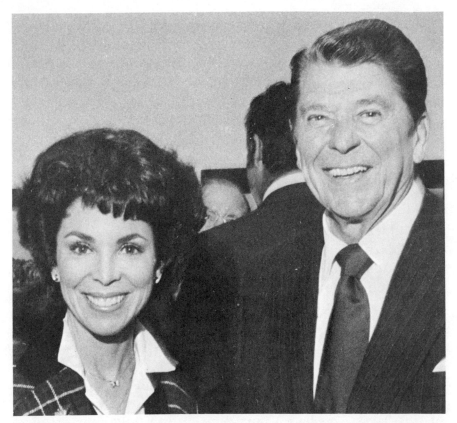

Author Maureen Salaman with President Ronald Reagan.

made *Public Scrutiny* the nation's leading pro-laetrile alternative therapy health news magazine and the magnifying glass for the medical consumers of America. In 1982, *Public Scrutiny's* name was changed to *Health Freedom News*.

By 1979, the case of Rutherford vs the FDA was fought through to the Supreme Court only to have that court deny the issues of constitutional freedom and right to privacy and remand it back to the Appellate Court to consider the "grandfathering issue".[1]

---

[1]*Grandfathering:* if a substance has been in common use prior to the establishment of the FDA, that agency must relinquish its authority over such. This book has more than established the fact of amygdalin grandfathering.

Predictably (though its line of reasoning boggles the mind), the Appellate Court denied the grandfathering of laetrile.

Thus a disheartening stalemate continues. The outlook is not brightened by the portent of many more months — perhaps years — of legal review and argument toward the sanctification, within the meaning of grandfathering, of amygdalin's already-established immunity from FDA regulation — let alone FDA harrassment of doctors using amygdalin in an effort to save lives. Amygdalin was here, and in use, long before the FDA was created. No amount of time-consuming litigation can alter that fact.

It is ludicrous in the extreme, then, that this issue, as the crux of the Rutherford case, should have had to be dragged through a series of lengthy, costly and unnecessary court actions in the first place. Again, the people lose. (Big Brother, you see, has prostituted the powers we have vested in him by misusing them to abridge our constitutionally-guaranteed rights.)

So, in essence, we are forced to fight for something that is already ours. But we will continue to do so. It has been the remarkable spirit of the American people that has thus far sustained us in this battle for the vindication of laetrile amygdalin therapy. With their continuing dedication, the temporary setback of this latest Appellate Court decision can only spur us on to renewed, concerted legislative effort on the national level.

United action on such a scale, needless to say, is financially costly. Unfortunately, no person, no organization, is blessed with the vast resources it takes to prevail against the tax-supported legal might of the FDA, buttressed by the enormous funds of the orthodox medical establishment. But, as we have already pointed out, there is strength in numbers — in which, fortunately, we the people have a tremendous edge. Contributions, no matter how small or large, will provide the collective financial clout needed to assure victory for both the amygdalin forces and the thousands upon thousands of cancer victims they represent.

But who can best utilize these funds toward a triumphant campaign? Which organization, of all those in the pro-amygdalin camp, is best structured in people and operational machinery to implement such a massive effort most effectively and productively? There are a number of selfless cancer-fighting entities, already mentioned in this book's preceding pages. And while each of them could use every dollar they can muster, their individual efforts could, at best, constitute a fragmentary, rather than unified, attack.

There is one, however, that is capable of marshalling and applying the combined strength of all cancer-fighting amygdalin supporters in a solid, unbeatable front. That organization is the National Health Federation.

The NHF, 40,000 members strong, is already committed to an all-out effort. Its legal counsel is exceptionally well-qualified (and extensively experienced through previous encounters with the federal bureaucracy) to combat the anti-freedom-of-choice forces in Washington and other sectors of the establishment. The NHF has great respect for, and has worked closely with, other cancer-fighting entities; many of its members are also supporters of these organizations and have made contributions to them in the past. Now, however, they recognize the NHF as the strongest single body to champion the cause of all. At this point, it is hoped, you are of the same persuasion.

On that assumption, the following answer is proposed to the question you are undoubtedly asking as you read this: "What can I do to help?" By all means, give your support, in whatever amount you can afford, to the NHF. Without in any way disparaging the original ideals and aims of the American Cancer Society or those of the truly public-spirited organizations named in the Foreword to this book, the authors offer their fullest assurance that under the efforts and auspices of the NHF, the dollars you contribute to its ever-growing fund could not possibly be used with more telling effect in meeting our mutual commitment to the eradication of cancer in our lifetime.

The choice is yours, of course (and it is that very freedom that inspired this book if you will recall). The only decision you have to make is who can best make your check work for the greatest good. That should be easy, if you already happen to be a member of the

National Health Federation. If not, you might be left to wonder whether your support should pay for television spots imploring viewers to "get a check-up and give a check" or be used more appropriately to gain the legalization of natural therapies that could free humanity forevermore from the scourge of cancer.

Readers wishing to send contributions to the NHF cancer legislation fund should make checks payable to the National Health Federation. All such contributions are tax-deductible. Please address all correspondence to: National Health Federation, Cancer Fund, 212 West Foothill Boulevard, Monrovia, CA 91016. Due to the vast number of letters received, NHF cannot make personal acknowledgements to every donor, but names and the amounts of contributions will be recorded in NHF publications as an expression of gratitude for the support given to this worthy cause.

In supporting the NHF, you will be putting your money on a winner. Because this is one fight the NHF does not intend to lose — not only against cancer, but for the perpetuation of your right to a freedom of choice in the measures by which you (all of us) maintain optimum health. Together, we can serve no higher purpose.

APPENDIX III:

Faulty Testing of Laetrile

The medical and governmental forces to this day intentionally misinform the public and, worse, thwart all efforts to apply nutrtional therapy to the prevention and mitigation of cancer. Let us look at some historical background.

On April 30, 1981, at a meeting of the Society of Clinical Oncology in Washington, D.C., Charles Moertel, M.D., of the Mayo Clinic presented the following conclusion, drawn from his Phase II study* of laetrile authorized by the National Cancer Institute:

"Laetrile has been tested — it is not effective."

It is the contention of every recognized laetrile authority that the substance Dr. Moertel tested in this Phase II test was not, in fact, laetrile; rather it was a degraded substance, the molecular structure of which differed substantially from that of naturally-occurring laetrile amygdalin. The following facts have been established: 1) the NCI and full knowledge that the material they specified for the test did not meet the biochemical specifications of amygdalin as defined by the federal courts, as listed in all the medical journals and pharmacopoeias, and as used in all the previous successful laboratory and clinical evaluations; 2) the NCI's *own* test medical director, Dr. Moertel, had, prior to commencing the Phase II tests, voiced his opposition to using the so-called laetrile provided by the NCI.

---

*After the previous Phase I test Dr. Moertel had stated unequivocally that laetrile, or amygdalin, was non-toxic when taken in normally prescribed amounts.

It is important — indeed, a life-and-death matter for many present and future cancer patients — that an unbiased examination of the facts in this matter be made, for two reasons. First to ascertain whether or not genuine laetrile was ever tested. Second, to arrive at a judgment as to whether the negative statement of Dr. Moertel was, or was not, supported by incontestable scientific proof.

This book, in production before the NCI tests were completed, repeatedly emphasizes how vitally important it is to understand that laetrile amygdalin is therapeutically effective only when administered *in its natural form*. A definitive explanation of why only natural amygdalin has therapeutic value is contained in the compendium of E. T. Krebs, Jr., (the discoverer and co-developer of laetrile amygdalin) included in this book's Appendix.

A historical review of the laetrile movement provides this interesting revelation: In 1970, the McNaughton Foundation (the leader for over a quarter-century in sponsoring the orderly development of laetrile through both scientific research and in unending dialogue with establishment medical, scientific, and political interests) filed for and was granted I.N.D. (investigational new drug) Permit #6734 for a Phase II (Phase II test is commenced only after it is proved conclusively in a Phase I test that the subject material is non-toxic in prescribed amounts) trial of laetrile amygdalin; this permit, for what appears to be political reasons, was rescinded less than 10 days after its issuance.

In December, 1979, Permit #16013 was granted to the NCI — also for a Phase II study of amygdalin. However, the molecular structure of the amygdalin for which the permit was issued was substantially different from that specified for the originally-proposed trial. We ask the reader: How can the Food and Drug Administration (FDA) explain issuing two permits for the clinical testing of laetrile where the materials to be used in each of the two tests did not have identically the same technical specifications?

Was this the result of an unscientific (even if subconscious) desire on the part of the NCI for the tests to fail? Reference to correspondence between the Mayo Clinic and the McNaughton Foundation, prior to the government-sponsored tests, can lead to no other conclusion.

Let's look back now to December of 1978. By this point in time over 20 states had, without precedence, granted their citizens the freedom of choice to use nontoxic holistic laetrile therapy in the treatment of their cancers. Bowing to this political pressure, plus a Federal Court decision allowing the importation and interstate shipment of amygdalin, the NCI filed an investigational new drug application for the testing of laetrile.

The scientific closed-mindedness with which the testing of laetrile was approached — and the preconcluded and ordained result — may be discerned from a statement, quoted in *Newsweek* magazine, by no less than Dr. Vincent DeVita, NCI's Director of Cancer Research: "If people have to have clinical tests carried out in order to prove to them that laetrile doesn't work, maybe we will have to do it that way."

When the original protocol (design and specifications) for the proposed test first appeared, the entire leadership of the laetrile movement protested that the material NCI proposed to test was not laetrile. Spearheading this protest were the Cancer Control Society, the International Association of of Cancer Victims and Friends, the National Health Federation, the McNaughton Foundation, the Nutrisearch Foundation, and all of the scientific and medical advocates of laetrile therapy. Included in this latter group were Dr. E. T. Krebs, Jr., laetrile's co-discoverer, and Dr. Dean Burk, former head of cyto-chemistry at the NCI.

The following headline appeared in the July, 1980, issue of *Public Scrutiny,* a publication of the National Health Federation: ARE THE NATIONAL CANCER INSTITUTE CLINICAL TRIALS WITH LAETRILE FOREDOOMED TO FAILURE? The article thereunder concludes as follows:

"The result of using DL-amygdalin in place of D-amygdalin would prove nothing one way or another about the efficacy of Laetrile. Such spurious tests would be a sad waste of time and public money."

Let us re-emphasize that this outcry against the material specified by NCI began more than a year prior to the test commencement and it came from both professional and lay advocates of laetrile, with one exception, unfortunately, a Mr. Robert Bradford. This entrepreneur, trading on his influence as a former president of the Committee for Freedom of Choice, contacted directors of NCI and persuaded them to specify a Mexican material for which, not so oddly enough, he happened to be the major distributor.

Mr. Bradford was, at the time, well aware that the material he distributed did not meet the identification specification for natural, therapeutically-active amygdalin.[1] However, Mr. Bradford represented in literature, correspondence, and personal conversation with NCI that the unnatural conformation of the product he sold was the result of "a manufacturing process in common use" and that "any alteration of that process would be in conflict with the good manufacturing practice code of the F.D.A."[2] He further stated (in knowing opposition to all recognized laetrile authorities, not the least of whom was Dr. Krebs) that "nothing in the literature or theory substantiated that epimerization (the changing of natural amygdalin to an unnatural form) affected its therapeutic efficacy."[3]

It is pertinent to note here that Mr. Bradford's sole income at the time was derived from selling a product represented to be laetrile amygdalin, which was actually (as he has since acknowledged) subpotent and degraded.[4] Despite this fact, or because of it, the NCI was given, by Mr. Bradford, an excuse to use an injectable substance of such questionable therapeutic merit that only a test result matching their preconceived determination of failure could have been arrived at. The final NCI test protocol specified the use of a natural amygdalin in tablet form and an unnatural liquid amygdalin unequivalent to technical specifications, for injection. Such inconsistency is considered, throughout the scientific community, to be professionally unpardonable.

Following is a condensation of correspondence between the McNaughton Foundation and the Mayo Clinic prior to the test (note the writer's apprehension):

6 Feb 79

To: Dr. Charles Moertel
    Mayo Clinic

Dear Dr. Moertel:

In a spirit of sincerity and cooperation I would like to offer some comments with respect to your proposed clinical protocols.

In a letter from the F.D.A. to N.C.I. I am concerned to note that the material intended for use as injection is the unnatural DL-amygdalin.

All of the Laetrile-amygdalin in use prior to 1971 was the D-isomer as found in nature (R configuration). This was in accord with both Krebs and Merck Index specifications. Subsequent to 1971, after the withdrawal of our I.N.D. #6734, production of Laetrile in California was terminated.

Sometime in 1972 or 1973 production of Laetrile was taken over by a Mexican corporation, which for various reasons, and against our repeated and continued objections, commenced to supply unnatural DL-amygdalin in their injectable vials.

All of the pioneering animal and clinical work with Laetrile amygdalin was carried out with the pure natural D-amygdalin.

The unnatural DL-amygdalin has been distributed only since 1974 when production of Laetrile in the U.S.A. and Canada ended.

The excellent therapeutic results achieved clinically with pure natural D-amygdalin were obtained with doses fractionally smaller than with the impure Mexican product, presently being distributed in the United States.

I am enclosing Xerox copies of authoriative works on amygdalin. You will readily   see that the use of unnatural racemic DL-amygdalin in the coming trials can only confuse an understanding of any clinical result and, most certainly, not be acceptable as a true evaluation of the potential of Laetrile therapy for cancer.

Sincerely,

A. McNAUGHTON
McNaughton Foundation

Included in the works sent to both Mayo and the NCI was the compendium of Krebs' papers on therapeutic amygdalin, published by the Nutrisearch Foundation, and included in Appendix VII of this book. Before we present Dr. Moertel's reply to Mr. McNaughton, it is important to clarify the therapeutic differences between amygdalin and its unnatural, degraded, counterpart involved in this controversy.

The product D-amygdalin (laetrile) is pure amygdalin, unchanged from its biochemical state in the living plant; DL-amygdalin is not laetrile but *was* amygdalin in the living plant. In the process of extraction and packaging, DL-amygdalin becomes denatured (subject to intramolecular changes) and thus deviates from anything common to biological experience. The denaturation of the molecule converts it from amygdalin (laetrile — a nutrient) to a drug. As such, DL-amygdalin has no counterpart in living plants and, as an adulterated substance, is devoid of any therapeutic activity. It was this later adulterated substance NCI specified for Dr. Moertel to test.

Feb 14 1979

To: McNaughton Foundation
      San Ysidro, CA
From: Mayo Clinic
Dear Mr. McNaughton:

I am very grateful for your letter of February 6th. We had received correspondence from Mr. Robert Bradford stating there was no evidence that one form of amygdalin was superior to another. *Based on this information it had been our intent to use the racemic DL-amygdalin. Based on your letter I have conveyed to the National Cancer Institute my recommendation that the natural D form be prepared for intravenous use. This will result in a substantive delay in initiating the trials but I feel it is most important to do this properly.* [Italic ours.]

Sincerely,

DR. CHARLES MOERTEL, M.D.
Mayo Clinic

Between Dr. Moertel's February 14 and March 16 letters, a significant change occurred. In the following letter, Dr. Moertel refers to what is in current use, rather than what is scientifically correct. The material advocated by laetrile's developers and pioneering clinicians was already destined, by higher authority, to be ignored. The NCI had no doubt informed him they intended to supply only material identical to the substandard Mexican material submitted to them by Mr. Bradford. (He was, remember, this material's major distributor.)

March 16, 1979

To: McNaughton Foundation
From: Mayo Clinic

Dear Mr. McNaughton:

I wish to thank you for your recent correspondence regarding the proposed clinical trials of Laetrile.

Analyses conducted by the National Cancer Institute as well as by independent laboratories have indicated that the material proposed for intravenous use is identical to that which is *currently* being used by Laetrile practitioners. The National Cancer Institute and Mr. Robert Bradford have recently arranged for an exchange of material.

We have made every effot to conform to the metabolic and dietary program supplied to us by Mr. Bradford.

Sincerely,

CHARLES G. MOERTEL, M.D.
Mayo Clinic

Every laetrile scientist, without exception, abhorred the quality of laetrile produced in Mexico (for which, in addition to being its distributor, Mr. Bradford claimed to be the quality consultant.[5]) Several previously published studies by FDA laboratories stated that Mr. Bradford's Mexican material was not only adulterated, it was subpotent as well, and did not even meet the technical specification for amygdalin.[6]

The fact that the NCI would accept the very specification of amygdalin they had previously condemned — at the recommendation of its major distributor — is scientifically and rationally incomprehensible.

Mr. McNaughton noted this reversal of intent to use natural amygdalin for injection. In the following letter, he again re-emphasizes the unanimity of laetrile authorities and requests Dr. Moertel to think about the implication of using substandard material that the NCI was evidently intent upon supplying.

26 March 1979

From: McNaughton Foundation
To: Mayo Clinic
Dear Dr. Moertel:

Thank you so much for your letter of March 16, 1979. Perhaps I have misunderstood your letter but I am under the impression that the implication of your second paragraph is that the injectable Laetrile now to be used in the clinical trials will not be pure natural amygdalin.

It would be a mistake to use a DL mixture in the coming trials in place of the single D isomer of amygdalin as found in nature and as described in the Merck Index and elsewhere. After all, iso-amygdalin and neo-amygdalin are no the same as amygdalin....

Sincerely,

ANDREW L. McNAUGHTON

In a final letter to the McNaughton Foundation, Dr. Moertel absolves himself of any obligation to use true amygdalin in the proposed tests. In so doing, he places full responsibility for any prospect of failure on the NCI and on the recommendation and information given them by Mr. Bradford.

January 9, 1980

Mr. Andrew L. McNaugton
THE McNAUGHTON FOUNDATION
PO Box B-17
San Ysidro, California 92073
Dear Mr. McNaughton:

I have passed on all of your recommendations for change in the clinical protocol and I hope that most of these will be adopted. I, of course, have had no direct role in drug formulation which is being carried out entirely by the National Cancer Institute. [Italics ours.]

Sincerely,

CHARLES C. MOERTEL, M.D.
Mayo Clinic

CGM: mab
Enclosures

Copies of all the preceding correspondence were sent to the National Cancer Institute as well as all major laetrile advocates. It is abundantly clear that the NCI, in 1979 (prior to commencing the Phase II tests), knew the material they proposed to use was improper by their own previous tests,[7] by the opinion of the doctor they had designated to supervise the test, and by every legitimate laetrile advocate except the world's largest distributor of Mexican material.[8]

Just as logic based on a false assumption leads to a false conclusion, so any test program based upon an incorrect substance will inevitably yield a false result. The facts in this case bear incontestable testimony (albeit regrettable!) to the soundness of this fundamental scientific axiom. Let us review them in order.

Fact: The material administered did not match the technical specifications for therapeutic natural amygdalin.

Fact: A Phase II test of any anti-tumoral substance is defined by NCI as primarily judgmental of tumor reduction; but, as this book explains, tumor reduction is not the immediately desired result of nutritionally oriented laetrile therapy.

Fact: The quantities of both enzymes and vitamins given during this test were highly questionable.

Fact: The patients chosen for the study were all patients who, to quote NCI, "had proven cancer beyond hope of cure," and whose immune system had already been irreparably destroyed.

Fact: Patients who showed even headaches were immediately removed from the program and became a negative statistic. (Although the FDA ignores the devastating side effects of conventional radiation and chemotherapy treatments.)

Fact: Even the degraded DL material administered was in far smaller amounts than called for in the original protocol.

Fact: The authorized double blind study on palliation never even began.

Given all these precursors of failure, what other result could the trial tests possibly have had? That they proved negative is academic in light of the principal and overriding fact that the correct therapeutic D-amygdalin was not used in the first place. This was true not only of the injectable amygdalin, but also of the tablets, which independent laboratory analysis have since shown to also be iso-amygdalin. If anything at all was proved, it was that even molecularly degraded amygdalin is nontoxic; and further, that the material used produced no better results (but certainly no worse) than the 30-or-so approved drugs — many of which are violently toxic — that had previously been used without beneficial results on the patients subjected to the test.

We wish to cast no aspersions upon the many fine oncologists who conducted these tests unaware that what they were testing was not laetrile amygdalin. We do believe, however, that it was incumbent upon Dr. Moertel to include in his press packet, as is customary, the technical specifications of the materials used in the test and to acknowledge, furthermore, the opinion of laetrile advocates and scientists that the material used was actually a non-therapeutic, unnatural form of amygdalin.

Perhaps Dr. Moertel was influenced by the commercial audacity of Mr. Bradford who in the spring of 1980 switched from his Mexican source to distributing the amygdalin of another manufacturer and subsequently sued Mayo Clinic, Dr. Moertel, NCI, et al., to prevent the tests from continuing with the material he had recommended in the first place.[9] Such hyprocrisy, no doubt, was the thorn that festered and ultimately — to the detriment of many now-deprived cancer victims — influenced Dr. Moertel to question the integrity of the entire laetrile movement. Of such stuff are tragedies made!

So much, then, for history. And for the injustices that inspired the writing of this book. But truth will out. What we know of it is presented throughout this treatise as objectively as possible, without fear or favor, in the interest of clearing the air on the controversial subject of cancer. Many issues remain unsolved. But as you read on, solutions to the mysteries of cancer will become apparent. Chief among them are guidelines based on the conviction that you need never fall victim to this dread disease if you follow the course of prevention through nutrition. This is the area where naturally occurring amygdalin, is destined to make its greatest contribution in the decade of the '80s.

As Dr. Krebs, Jr., has stated so aptly, "We have been brought to the realization that in the national management of cancer we are dealing with a problem of nutrition; and nutrition never has been, or is today, a part of crisis medicine. We are dealing with a vitamin. Therefore we will not be bound by the conventions of crisis medicine."

And that is the crux of the issue, as viewed by advocates of laetrile amygdalin: whether to permit conventions and hyprocrisy to stifle all hope of conquering cancer, or to fight for the freedom to attack it with the most effective weapons at our command. Amygdalin may not be the final answer. But it is, at this writing, the best weapon we have, when used in conjunction with the program offered here. That it has not been legalized nationally in the United States is both a medical and moral calamity. until that time comes, the reader is urged to evaluate the preventive approaches outlined in this book and follow his own conscience.

It is encouraging, meanwhile, that more and more Americans — led by people in high office — are rallying to the cause around which this whole controversy rages: the right to choose one's own destiny. Perhaps most important are the substantively identical statements of the presidential Press Secretary, speaking for President Reagan when informed of the Mayo test results, and of Governor Jay Rockefeller upon signing, the following day, a laetrile freedom bill for West Virginia (making it the 25th state to do so): "What the test proves or disproves is not important. What is important is the right of every American citizen to freedom and choice in matters of health."

Readers of this book do, in a sense, have a choice. One is to risk becoming one of the 1-in-4 Americans destined to contract cancer and then receive the crisis treatments offered by the orthodox medical establishment. The other is to follow the herein-outlined plan of nutrition recommended by a new generation of preventive medicine physicians — and thus free themselves from the menace of this devastating degenerative disease.

Beyond that, we can be guided by our faith in the ultimate power of the people to prevail over government demagoguery. As

William Blake said of America in a statement made in 1817, which still rings true today: "Tho obscured, this is the form of the angelic land." If only Americans could understand, once again, the potential for tyranny that exists as long as federal agencies continue to proliferate their power to tell us what to put in our mouths!

If we can recognize that fact and rise to the challenge, we can not only defeat political oppression but, in the process, rid ourselves of cancer — once and for all. Together, with faith in God and the principle right that makes might, "We have it in our power," as Thomas Paine wrote in *Common Sense* in 1776, "to begin the world again."

Notes — APPENDIX III

1. Technical Identification Specifications for Amygdalin Laetrile, 10th Federal District Court, Judge Bohannon; IS-630-RO. Published by Bradford Foundation.
2. Ibid.
3. "The Metabolic Management of Cancer," The Robert Bradford Foundation, Los Altos, CA, 1979.
4. *Choice* Magazine, Spring and Summer, 1980, Los Altos, CA.
5. "Now That You Have Cancer," Choice Publications, Inc. Los Altos, CA, 1977.
6. Cancer Treatment Reports, vol. 62:1, January, 1978.
7. Thomas Cairns, et al., John K. Howie and D. T. Sawyer, U.S. Food and Drug Administration, Los Angeles, CA 90015.
8. American Biologics advertisements, *Let's LIVE* Magazine, 1979.
9. *Choice* Magazine, Spring and Summer, 1980, Los Altos, CA.

APPENDIX IV:

A Trident Attack Against the Government/Medical/ Industrial Combine

Many individuals recognize the deliberate obstructionism and apathy toward preventive, holistic, and nutritional medicine presented by the orthodox establishment. They consider these problems so massive and overwhelming, however, that these obstructions can only be overcome by the institution of vast government programs that, in and of themselves, act to stifle creative medicine.

We have referred throughout this book to a governmental/ industrial/medical combine. Drug companies could never have achieved a stranglehold over the health of the American public without the implementation of government force.

One must draw the distinction between competitive free, private enterprise, the most moral and productive system ever devised, and cartel capitalism, dominated by industrial monopolists, international bankers and their government sycophants. Private enterprise operates by offering products, therapies, and services in a competitive free market. From such competition the consumer gets the best product for the lowest price. The moment the quality of a merchant's product or service is not the best or his price becomes too high, he will lose business to a competitor. Problem solving in a free enterprise society is accomplished by the profit incentive. Wherever there is a profit to be made by providing superior service an entrepreneur will supply the need with the consumer patient becoming the ultimate benefactor. Conversely, cartel capitalists or monopolistic capitalists use government, and its restrictive legislation, bureaus (FDA/USDA) licensing requirements, to force the public to do business with them alone. Cartel capitalists are the deadly enemies of competitive private enterprise. These combinations and their use of government power have enabled establishment medicine and the drug industry to prevent innovative new techniques and therapies.

This is nothing less than corporate socialism. We must resist the urge to call in the very government which caused the problem in the first place. Various people of good intent have suggested solutions to our nutritional and medical dilemmas which consist of redistribution of farm land, more stringent regulations on the drug industry and a myriad of well-meaning, high-sounding do-good governmental programs.

Inherent in the execution of such programs is the tenent that in order for the government to grant privilege to one group of citizens it must reduce the freedom inherent in the balance of its population. This, of course, is always financed through taxing away from certain citizens that which they rightfully earned and deserve to keep. As this confiscation escalates, incentive is destroyed and more and more people look to government to provide for them, never realizing that government produces nothing; it can only continue to confiscate a portion of the increasingly shrinking production of its citizens.

Nowhere in the history of the human race is there any justification for the naive faith in political power that is bedrock thinking of those who proffer collectivist solutions to all our medical problems in the form of ever-increasing government influence, regulations, and the size of the bureaucratic establishment.

We have been continually lulled by the lie that "Washington can do it for us" or "we can depend on the government to look out for our best interests." In order to believe that, one must presume that government possesses a superior wisdom that individual citizens do not. After so many years of experience with officialdom, Americans should know that government agencies are not repositories of infinite wisdom. One need only watch an Ehrlichman doing a Watergate to see the fallacy of such an assumption.

The oft-repeated phrase, "we are the government," is naive at best in light of the facts.

The reins of government power have been taken from the hands of the people, and are now being dispensed by an unconstitutional, unelected, unresponsive fourth branch of the federal government. The Food and Drug Administration (FDA) is a prime example. Its sovereignty does not constitute rule by law where the people keep legitimate restraints on government. It constitutes rule by decree — the decree of federal regulatory agencies. We have lost more freedom through these agencies than by all the Acts of Congress combined.

One of the most important aspects of state legalization of laetrile is in showing people their way back to freedom. Citizens are exerting their rights over the Washington bureaucrats, telling them to keep hands off the sovereignty each individual should rightly possess over his or her body.

The Tenth Amendment of the Constitution ensures our freedom. Simply stated, it says to government, "Anything we forgot, you can not do that either." Whether we realize it or not, we are presently experiencing the result of our past choices. Your tomorrow depends upon your choices today. Once the people realize they can control and reduce the power of these federal agencies, not only will the new theories of medicine and nutrition be available to choose or reject by an informed community, but other freedoms will be regained as well.

Court rulings, such as the Bohannon Decision on laetrile, can solve some problems, but the final solution is to dismantle the power structure within these agencies. This requires congressional action responding to the desires of the electorate. An example of enlightened legislation is a bill by Congressman Larry McDonald of Marietta, Georgia, which would take away the FDA's power to rule on the efficacy of a drug and confine their regulatory authority to the area of dangerous toxicities.

In 1962, because of the thalidomide scare, the Harris-Kefauver amendment gave the FDA purview over the efficacy of a new drug. The FDA at that time already had the power to stop thalidomide because they had purview over dangerous drugs; they actually covered up their own incompetent failure by requesting and gaining even more restrictive controls.

Certainly all consumers want drugs to be effective. But who has a greater stake in whether a drug is effective or not — a doctor who can empirically judge the results his patient receives, or a bureaucrat who has, at best, a passing or mild interest? Further, since the enactment of Harris-Kefauver, giving the FDA exclusive power to determine a drug's effectiveness, the time required for new drug approval has gone from 1-2 years to 10-12 years. Americans suffer, are crippled, and die from a multitude of diseases which can be treated and cured all over the world but not here in the United States of America, where restrictive bureaucracy prohibits the implementation of their curative modality. The cost of getting a new drug approved has gone from $1.2 million to from $14 million to $52 million, an insurmountable financial barrier to all but the giant drug conglomerates who thus perpetuate their monopoly.

In the *Congressional Record*, June 28th, 1976, Steve Symms stated, "In the last analysis, we are weighing loss of human lives. How many lives are lost because available therapy is bad or how many lives are lost because therapy is not available?"

An article entitled "The FDA Is Dangerous To Your Health," by William Hoar, published in *American Opinion* magazine in December, 1976, makes this disturbing observation: "You could die needlessly while the FDA fiddles. Had penicillin, aspirin, digitalis and insulin been introduced after 1962, they would have been banned by current Food and Drug Administration standards. So bad is the situation that three-fourths of the new U.S. drugs are prohibited here but used overseas."

A 1970 pre-inflationary study estimates that the 1962 efficacy drug amendment cost consumers, on balance, between $300 million and $400 million during 1970. The average amount of paperwork has gone from 75 pages before 1962 to 75,000 pages after 1962. This means that under the present stipulations we will not have another new natural substance such as laetrile, because no one will be willing to invest money in a substance which is in the public domain and therefore cannot be patented in order that investors can retrieve their investment.

So what can we do to correct this sorry state of affairs? The solution to the problem is three-pronged. First, the control of the government is still in the Congress. Let your congressman know that you want him to start slicing away at the tyrannical power structure of the FDA and other federal regulatory agencies to the extent that you are prepared, if need be, to support his opponent in the next election financially. The way to limit the power of these agencies is to elect congressmen who understand the potential for tyranny within these illegal, unconstitutional agencies. Or to at least make your existing congressman understand the gravity of the situation. If this fails, support congressman in other districts who have exhibited an understanding of the threat to life and liberty inherent in the fourth branch of government in general, and to the 1962 Harris-Kefauver Amendment in particular. You have the backing of the man upstairs, President Ronald Reagan, on this.

Second, educate the people around you, keeping in mind that we need companions — in what Jefferson referred to as "the holy cause of freedom" — not disciples. Stockholm's *Dagens Nyheter* observed, "Americans are not bound together by social and cultural ties, family or even language, so much as by the American dream itself."

In commenting on the American Revolution, the *London Sunday Telegram* confirmed that were it not for the "American Experiment" the idea of individual freedom would never have survived the 19th Century. The American experiment was consciously conceived as a momentous step in the evolution of the species. "The cause of America is in great measure the cause of all mankind."

Third, use your dollars as you would your vote. Support those merchants who give you wholesome, non-additive, organic foods and supplements, and withold your vote from those who do not, letting them know why. Once again, with sufficient education, the transgressors will not stay in business.

All this may seem like an impossible task. Each of us is only one. But we *are* one, and one, and one. In collective action, we take on the strength of the tide. And remember, to do nothing as individuals is to invite upon all of us as a whole the very fate we want so desperately to escape — and to be forevermore enslaved to the enemies of personal freedom.

APPENDIX V:

The Beneficiaries: Patients of Unorthodoxy

Janet and Jerry Devine of Dowingtown, Pa., the parents of 3-year-old Chad Devine, responded to their son's complaints of a backache, which started in November of 1972, by treating it with aspirin and a heating pad advised by a local orthopedist. In January, 1973, they took Chad to Philadelphia Children's Hospital where tests were made the following February. The findings indicated that the spine was curving, prompting the diagnosis that Chad had a fractured vertebrae. He was placed in a body cast that month, but his condition was even worse when he was released.

Janet Devine fights back tears as she recounts her little boy's ensuing experience. "Well before he was seven years old, Chad was in screaming pain 16 out of every 24 hours. He had been diagnosed with everything from psychological problems (both his and his mother's) to being 'too lazy to walk straight'."

It was not until the summer of 1974 that Chad's condition was diagnosed as cancer of the spine, this following an operation extending from his skull to the 11th vertebra. Doctors at the Children's Hospital in Philadelphia said the tumor was inoperable. The seven-year-old was temporarily paralyzed from the operation, then underwent radiation, and had to be carried everywhere since he could hardly move. A cancer specialist suggested chemotherapy — but the Devines had already seen the results of toxic chemotherapy on young cancer patients at the hospital. "Each day one child died," Mrs. Devine recalls, "and one day two died. It was a chamber of horrors." But she was told only radiation or chemotherapy would have a chance at halting cancer's growth in her son.

Following a spirited argument with a hospital doctor in which she said she had decided she would not let Chad undergo chemotherapy, the physician said, "If that is the way you feel, get the kid out of here." She did. Chad was very sick — "practically a vegetable," in Mrs. Devine's words. "We had to carry him around everywhere. He was like a rag doll."

It was two months later when her sister-in-law told her about a man in her church who had been bedridden with lung cancer but who had so recovered following vitamin B17 (laetrile) treatment that he was up and around and able to go hunting. Mrs. Devine felt that at that point she had nothing to lose.

By March 1975 they had found a kindly local doctor able to start young Chad on oral doses of B17 tablets — since the memory of dying children and chemotherapy had made Chad react violently to needles. Within three weeks, the semi-paralyzed son, who had had to be carried everywhere, whose weight had been 42 lbs., and who had been practically unable to hold anything on his stomach, was able to make a long-awaited trip to Disneyland. Within three months he was going to school again, something he had been unable to do because of his continual pain and screaming. His pain went away — particularly remarkable for a nine-year-old who had needed Demerol every four hours, and even that dosage was not enough.

Over 18 months later, Chad was at 66 lbs. Though having earlier lost partial use of his fingers, he began to play baseball and swim. According to a neurologist this meant that the pressure on the spine had been reduced and the tumor was shrinking.

Chad Devine (who, in 1973 at age eight had been given two years at the most to survive) is now 15 years old, plays Little League baseball, owns two horses which he rides and cares for himself and describes himself as being in excellent health. His mother says, "We know now we did the right thing. It has all turned out so well, like coming out of a nightmare." Chad's illness has brought an upgrading of lifestyle to the whole family and as a result of the improved diet, Chad's brothers and sisters, ages 19, 12 and 11, and the whole family enjoy excellent health.

The Rev. Clifford Oden is a Baptist minister and the former head of Garland Bible College in Garland, Texas. He suspected the worst when, in 1970, he picked up his telephone to hear his doctor say in a strained tone, "I sure need to see you right away."

"The blood drained from my face and the strength went out of my hands," recalls Rev. Oden. "I could hardly drive my car to his office. His report was what I feared: cancer of the colon! The only hope was an immediate colostomy. No other alternative! The time schedule? Within a week! The prediction? Five years."

Fellow Christians from all over the country joined him in the prayer that God would enable him to learn something about the cancer mystery that would be a help to other people. Within hours, Rev. Oden felt that his supplications had been answered with a flood of literature about laetrile metabolic therapy. The result? Clifford decided to forsake orthodoxy and go the nutritional laetrile metabolic route.

To this date Rev. Oden has not had the surgery. Nine different physicians, all of them in good standing and some of them internationally famous, have confirmed that the malignancy does exist, but so far it has been controlled by natural means. Without surgery, without radiation, without chemotherapy.

In gratitude for the knowledge of what Rev. Oden feels is God's concern for the welfare of the whole person, including the body, he has written a book titled, *Thank God I Have Cancer!*

Lynda Vasaturo of Bensalen, Pa., is a chic, well-groomed 5′ 7″ woman with good skin and a striking shock of shoulder-length, thick black naturally wavy hair.

Her doctors were blunt. The 33-year old housewife, they said, would have to spend the rest of her days pumped with chemicals in a hospital room. She had one year to live. She would be unable to function as a mother to her two small children. The 5-inch swelling in her leg had been diagnosed as a blood clot.

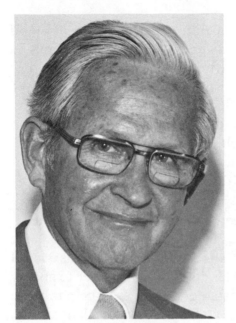

Rev. Clifford Oden

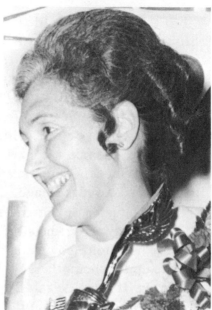

Carol Dunn

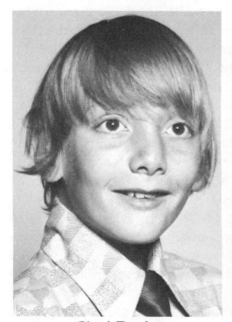

Chad Devine

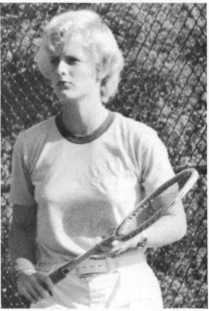

Chris Herbert

For three years, Lynda had been taking injections of blood thinners four times a week directly into the stomach (a terribly painful treatment). After detecting a lump in her stomach, she refused to take any more shots. Her doctors then operated and found a tumor 18 centimeters long. Lynda had obviously been treated for the wrong thing. Radiation treatments were begun, which Lynda recalls made her feel "like a piece of raw meat someone had poured boiling water over." She became sterile and went into radical change-of-life at only 29 years of age.

Two years later, she discovered a lump on the top of her head. The pathology report listed it as malignant. It was at this point that she was told how totally abnormal her functions would become under chemotherapy. Her doctors advised her to go buy marijuana. It wasn't legal, they stated, but it might help the side effects of the chemotherapy. The malignancy was back in her leg, left kidney, and was suspected in her liver.

It was at this point that Lynda decided to turn to laetrile metabolic therapy. If she was going to die, she decided to do it her way. How long she might live was of less concern to her than that she be able to live out of pain, care for her children and function as an otherwise normal human being. "I'm not going to lie down and be turned into a vegetable," she declared, "lose my hair and not be able to care for my children."

The New Jersey office of her physician, Dr. Cole, is exactly 53 miles from her home. Since starting laetrile nutritional therapy in 1978, she has driven there twice a week. Her objective response during this period has been that while her leg has been X-rayed, it is still the same; meanwhile, she has gone from 119 lbs. to 135 lbs. Her subjective response is that she feels great. She can not go skiing because her leg gives out (so much of the affected area was removed that the main blood vessels were cut away). Lynda, a pretty woman of wry good humor, reports her hair is again lovely and thick. When queried about her work level, she replied brightly, "I'm always active, I scrub my floors, go shopping, go to Disneyland on vacation. I'm on 6 grams of laetrile twice a week.

"I saw other people die," Lynda continued. "I had no faith in what the doctors were doing. It was very easy to try something else. My diet before had been Cheerios in the morning and sometimes Cream of Wheat; for lunch I would have white bread, peanut butter, soda and coke; for dinner, meat and boiled potatoes, canned vegetables and cake. The diet they put me on when I was on radiation consisted of beef, potatoes, all the milkshakes I could drink, no vegetables or seeds... that was the main thing and it only made me sicker.

"Now the whole family is on a new natural diet. This is the first year my 8-year-old daughter has not had allergies. Previously, it was nothing for Andrea to miss 45 days a year out of school; this year she has not missed a day. Valerie is 6. They are so much easier to live with now on our new diet."

If "tyranny, like hell, is not easily conquered," Carol Dunn gave her life's substance in the attempt. Carol, a striking woman with patrician features, lived 15 years beyond her death sentence. A former nurse, she was the winner of the coveted "Liberty Award," a woman of warmth, wit and an astute intellect. Her dedication, like that of Greg Kaye, can only be termed phenomenal.

Carol's immediate response, when the pathologist's report came back on July 8, 1965, "Lymphosarcoma and cancer of the bone marrow," was, "I have no time to die." In the 15 years that followed there was always one thing more Carol wanted to accomplish — and accomplish she did! She began radiation treatment. Her lymph nodes grew rapidly, particularly in the axillary area. The pain was considerable. Radiation seemed to increase the problem and Carol became convinced, by 1971, that is was the cause of the leukemia which had, by that time, appeared. It didn't take her long to decide to stop treatment.

In writing for *The Spotlight* (the nation's largest circulating individualist-constitutionalist newspaper), Carol first began to learn about, and subsequently speak and write on, alternative cancer approaches — from Charlotte Gerson Straus' therapy to germanium, spirogemanium, and Dr. Issel's therapy at the Ringberg Clinic in Rottach, Germany, to the laetrile therapy of Dr. Ray Evers. What she learned made an activist out of her and she was sure it would make an activist out of others.

Carol felt she could have been healed by these therapies, but by the time she found the truth on cancer cures, too much damage had been done by so-called "orthodox" doctors. Not only did Carol have no time to die, she had no time to spend on a complete cure.

She continued her relentless pace — many times showing up at her desk the morning after a lymph node had been surgically removed. By July, 1976, it had become an extreme effort for her to accomplish anything more strenuous than dictating articles from her bed. Much of her best work, ironically, was done when she was the most seriously ill. Her dream was to tell as many Americans as possible of the perils of orthodox cancer treatments. She wanted those who came after her to take her place in alerting the American people.

Carol's oncologist gave her an unlimited supply of the pain killer, percodan. The more she took, the more she needed. Soon no amount would stop the pain. A month of her life was lost in a mindless swirl of pain. Finally, with the help of Willis and Elizabeth Carto, she flew to Mexico and, mercifully, to laetrile treatment.

The first 10 days of her trip to Tijuana were a complete blank to her. She had to be carried in a wheelchair up the airport escalator in Los Angeles because the elevator was out of order. In San Diego, a forklift had to used to get her off the plane.

Finally, she was taken to her brother's house in Imperial Beach (just across the border from Tijuana). His wife, her sisters, and Elizabeth Carto took turns sleeping on the floor by her bed at night to comfort her and ration out her percodan. By the end of the month's treatment, the pain had completely subsided. Her energy returned. By April, she switched from intravenous laetrile to the tablets. She became ill with a rash and temperature.

After two days in the hospital and hundreds of tests at a cost of over $3,000, Carol was told she was allergic to oral tablets of laetrile. She continued to take injections 2 to 3 times a week. Carol, as a former nurse, considered the reaction no more severe than reactions in patients allergic to aspirin or penicillin — if, in fact, it was a reaction to laetrile, which she doubted. her reactions to chemotherapy and radiation were infinitely worse. In fact, actually life threatening.

The FDA released a warning on the purported laetrile allergic reaction without mentioning Carol's name. The spurious report was carried by the Associated Press and written up in the *Washington Post*. Carol, always rallying to the challenge, wrote a letter to the *Post* noting that while on laetrile her blood remained fairly stable. When she resorted to chemotherapy, the letter pointed out, her red blood count dropped from 28 to 23. The number of platelets in her bloodstream also dropped severely. Nor did chemotherapy reduce her enlarged lymph nodes.

She reminded the *Post* editors that at the present time she had the choice of taking full-body radiation (which could cause cancer in other parts of her body) or chemotherapy (which would cause nausea, vomiting, bone marrow depression, loss of hair, anemia, etc.). Could anyone honestly question her preference for laetrile, she asked?

Carol died on December 30, 1979, from pneumonia due to a weakened condition. She passed with the peace that surpasses understanding. In life she had looked forward with enthusiasm and anticipation to each new opportunity to serve — not for the glory it offered — but for the deep satisfaction of defending that which she so well knew to be right.

At this writing, Chris Herbert of East Brunswick, N.J., is 22. She has now been in remission from acute leukemia for several years. At age 12 she was diagnosed as having lymphoblastic leukemia. She went to New York for chemotherapy. She lost all her hair, lost her sense of balance and became practically an invalid. She was very weak. She suffered constant nausea, throwing up once a day. Her fever was 103° for one month. She could not keep food down.

Chemotherapy got her into remission but she contracted a bad infection from the chemotherapy which had to be operated on. She was on chemotherapy for one year. During that time she did not have more than four or five days functioning as a normal human being. She was an invalid, always ill. By October of 1974, Chris had left chemotherapy for treatment with Laetrile along with vitamins and enzymes. She noticed immediately that she was getting stronger and feeling better.

Chris is now on a tennis team and works managing her father's office. She is a tall, beautiful girl who is a glowing picture of health. She and her parents are great believers in Laetrile and metabolic therapy and work closely with Greg Kaye, the only legal Laetrile distributor in New Jersey, to get the message of Laetrile and metabolic therapy out to other people who are suffering the side effects of chemotherapy.

These are just five cases. There are many hundreds more, just as dramatic. To those of you who may think it strange in a book on cancer prevention case histories of cancer patients have been interjected, let me explain my reasoning.

I became involved in the natural approach to cancer to help a friend who was dying. Like Rev. Clifford Oden, Chad Devine, Lynda Vasaturo, Carol Dunn and Chris Herbert, I, too, at one time was a "junk food junkie" (Sara Lee was my patron saint!) I was sick without really being aware of it. I had lived with what I call "power outs" at approximately 4:00 p.m. for so long I accepted them as normal. It was when I actually began to witness, as it seemed to me, people being snatched from the jaws of death by simply changing their eating habits and adding supplementation that I became convinced that a change in nutrition offered the way to a more exuberant life for me. Since then I have experienced a threshhold of vitality, good health, and an abundance of energy and ambition I never realized existed.

I can offer you no greater gift than to share my good fortune with you. This has been my purpose in the writing of this book — for "Ye shall know the Truth and the Truth shall set you free."

The ultimate answer — the *only* answer to cancer — will be in prevention!

APPENDIX VI:

The Doctors

In spite of persecution that at times seemed to demonstrate a demonic zeal, doctors began to defect from the hallowed ranks of orthodoxy. Without exception they experienced first hand that the worst results obtainable with laetrile metabolic therapy in its optimum parameters are superior to the best results that strict orthodoxy has to offer.

The raison d'etre of the Laetrile Movement is that orthodoxy has failed. As this book has already illustrated, the incidence and death rates of cancer continue to increase with each passing year. The prevailing attitude of the non-orthodox forces is that of the over 1100 Americans who die of cancer each day most were hastened to their demise through the debilitating effects of the toxic orthodox modalities, a fact well documented in this book.

Among the defectors from orthodoxy is New York's Dr. Donald Cole. A visionary with the ability to focus in on the heart of a problem, Dr. Cole is a board-certified oncologist and former darling of the cancer establishment. As the recipient of an American Cancer Society fellowship at Memorial Sloan-Kettering, he was responsible for bringing some of the largest NCI grants in the country to St. Vincent's Hospital[1] of New York University. Most of the grants brought to St. Vincent's through Dr. Cole's genius and innovation are still there and the staff is continuing to perform these same tests even though they were proven unsuccessful years ago. Dr. Cole's wife, Barbara, a Cleopatra-type beauty with the face and figure of a China doll and an intellect as sharp as a laser beam, brings a tersely provocative light to the subject when she states, "If you had a cake recipe that did not work out and the cake fell, would you have 10 more people repeat it over and over?"

---

[1]St. Vincent's is among the world's largest hospitals.

Dr. Cole's interest in non-mutilating nutritional therapy evolved after many years of using traditional therapy where the tumor is the primary direction of all therapy. He explains that the patient therefore becomes secondary. "It is my feeling," he contends, "that if the therapy is curative then the side effect (toxicity) might be tolerable. But inasmuch as the therapy fails more often than it succeeds, a different approach must then be considered. I believe the therapy I now administer combines the best of all modalities. The results substantiate that side effects and toxicity and mutilation are not a necessary complement for a remission."

For Dr. Ray Evers, an early pioneer of metabolic therapy, the harrassment became so stifling that he fled to the Bahamas where he could enjoy a degree of freedom of the healing arts.

Considered by many the father of chelation therapy, he coined the word "wholistic", which means simply the treatment of the whole body. Dr. Evers has withstood 26 legal proceedings since 1974 at a cost to him in excess of $500,000. This makes this humanitarian doctor the most prosecuted and persecuted physician in the wholistic movement.

Dr. Evers now practices in Cottonwood, Alabama, where he is awaiting a decision of the Alabama Supreme Court on a five-year jail sentence resulting from a conviction on trumped up charges brought by a state narcotics agent who made it his special project to "get Dr. Evers" and dogged the 70-year-old physician's every move.

Dr. Harold Manner now has over 121 fully-staffed clinics using this therapy. The physicians who serve these clinics have been personally trained by Dr. Manner in an effort to control variables within the parameters of the testing. Included in the patient's data input is the name of the doctor who diagnosed the patient — how he was diagnosed, and the determination of the diagnosis. Every three-month period after the diagnostic tests are in, the patient is encouraged to take the results of these tests back to the doctor who first diagnosed him. The treating physician evaluates the results of these tests by checking one of a selection of four of the following choices:

1) Improved
2) No Improvement
3) Worse
4) Died

Well over 100 cases have already come in, as of this writing, and even though the state of the average patient is hopelessly terminal, the statistics are showing a 68 percent success rate.

James Privitera, M.D., practices in Covina, California. He is a licensed physician who received his M.D. degree from Creighton University School of Medicine in Omaha, Nebraska. Dr. Privitera interned at Providence Hospital in Seattle and at Presbyterian Hospital in San Francisco. In 1970, he entered private practice in allergy and nutrition. His practice led him to an interest in the properties of amygdalin in combination with enzymes and vitamin therapy. He was encouraged by the results he was getting. Then, in October 1974, he was given treatment ordinarily reserved for armed robbery suspects. Police arrested him in the middle of the night, put him in handcuffs and took him to jail on a conspiracy charge — conspiracy to prescribe an unapproved medicine. A Superior Court judge in San Diego threw that charge out of court. But the harrassment continued.

The State brought a second charge against Dr. Privitera and this time got a conviction and a sentence to six months in jail. In the 4th District Court of Appeals, Judge Robert Staniforth wrote a masterful opinion holding the California statute unconstitutional. The State appealed and Dr. Privitera lost 5-2 in the State

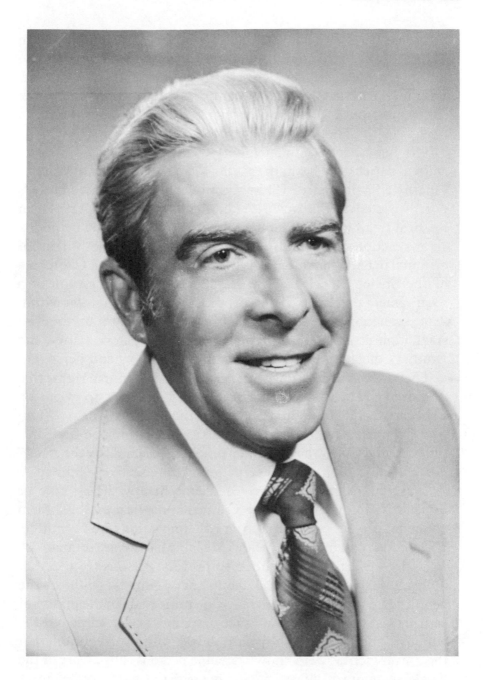

Dr. Harold Manner

Supreme Court. Chief Justice Rose Elizabeth Bird sided with Staniforth in her dissenting opinion, from which I quote: "So long as there is no clear evidence that Laetrile is unsafe to the user, I believe each individual patient has a right to obtain the substance from a licensed physician who feels it appropriate to prescribe it to him."

The issue here is human liberty. Can the informed cancer-ridden patient be limited to choice of treatments to "state-sanctioned" alternatives? The right to control one's own body is not restricted to the wise; it includes the "foolish" refusal of medical treatments. To require the doctor to use only orthodox state-sanctioned methods of treatment under the threat of criminal penalty for variance is to invite a repetition in California of the Soviet experience with Lysenkoism. The mention of a requirement that licensed doctors must prescribe and treat within "state-sanctioned" alternatives raises the specter of medical stagnation at best, and at worst, statism — paternalistic "Big Brother" dictating our options, both professional and personal.

The case was such a fundamental violation of human rights that it moved syndicated columnist James Kilpatrick to write on February 21, 1980 (quoted here from the *Sacramento Bee*: "This (the California law) is precisely the kind of statute one finds in a totalitarian regime, where medical practice is dictated by the state." Under California law, cancer patients are effectively limited to (1) surgery, (2) radiation or (3) chemotherapy. They may be hopelessly, terminally ill. The California medical establishment could not care less. No "unapproved" innovations are permitted. The wishes of an informed, knowledgeable patient are immaterial.

Up to a point, laws intended to prevent persons from acting foolishly may be tolerable. Beyond that point, the right of the people to be wrong must constantly be protected. In the matter of laetrile, California has tossed that fundamental principle out the window. The evidence in this case shows, without exception, that the cancer victims were knowledgeable persons fully aware of the "state-sanctioned" alternatives. These are not wide-eyed country bumpkins asking to be conned. They felt the imminency of death.

Both the court dissenters to the Privitera ruling and columnist Kilpatrick agreed that to imprison a doctor who is willing to try an unapproved medication with the consent of his patient reaches a "new depth of inhumanity." Rose Bird, herself a cancer victim who had experienced a mastectomy, said, "I cannot for the life of me comprehend the cruelty of the California law."

Jim served three months of his six months sentence doing hard labor. As this book goes to press, California has adopted an emasculated law which would permit oncologists in a research institution to use laetrile (none are, to your author's knowledge).

Governor Jerry Brown's office was inundated with petitions generated by Dr. Privitera's wife, Roseanne. Working in conjunction with the NHF she stumped the state rallying the people of the state to demand a pardon for James Privitera. Jim's parole board had voted 6 to 2 to pardon the good doctor. Through all this, Jim's wife sparked the conscience of a nation. She worked tirelessly, guesting on radio, telling her story in news articles and on TV shows throughout the state, eloquently denouncing "an atrocity of such magnitude that it cries our for vengeance."

Finally, on Friday, January 22, 1982, Governor Brown announced at the Long Beach convention of the National Health Federation that he had pardoned Dr. Privitera. A step on the side of righteousness, to be sure. And one for which the doctor's supporters are understandably grateful. But has right actually triumphed? A pardon carries the implication — and stigma — of initial guilt. Was one of society's laws breached or was Dr. Privitera working for society's good by invoking, in the highest sense of medical propriety, a right (if not a humanitarian's obligation to his conscience) fully guaranteed by law in 27 other states of this Union?

The pardon, unfortunately, does not expunge the record, as would a U.S. Supreme Court decision overturning the State Supreme Court's ruling. Nor does it compensate Jim Privitera for the loss, during the period of his incarceration, of the income that would have been his otherwise, his legal expenses or the cost of maintaining his professional facilities and the goodwill built up over a long period of service to his community.

The scar is still there, and always will be, just as much as one left by a careless surgeon who removes a perfectly healthy organ by mistake. The ultimate tragedy and irony in the Privitera case is that not only he, but perhaps hundreds of desperate cancer victims as well, have been deprived. They have been deprived by order of the state, not by the will of the people the state is honor-bound to serve, nor by the will of the Almighty who gave us our life-sustaining source of amygdalin.

There can be no adequate redress for the wounds inflicted upon Jim Privitera, a fine doctor who has, on behalf of all of us, borne the cross of man's inhumanity to man. One can only hope that, in time, those who forced him to bear it will themselves be seen as the betrayers, and made to suffer the opprobrium of an enlightened electorate that shows the good sense to replace them with men of vision and moral integrity.

Perhaps justice will one day be served in this case. Meanwhile, the wrong done Dr. James Privitera and the sanctity of our constitutional guarantee of freedom of choice remains on the record, unrequited. The issue — while our citizenry sleeps and thousands of cancer victims die needlessly — remains unresolved.

How much longer can we, the American people, afford to leave it at that?

APPENDIX VII:

The Extraction, Identification and Packaging of Therapeutically Effective Amygdalin

Extracted from a compendium of papers
written by Dr. E. T. Krebs, Jr.
co-discoverer and developer of Laetrile-amygdalin,
for the John Beard Memorial Foundation

THE INFORMATION CONTAINED HEREIN IS OF VITAL IMPORTANCE TO ALL MEDICAL PERSONNEL WHO WISH TO OBTAIN THE FULL CLINICAL POTENTIAL OF AMYGDALIN THERAPY

"Words can conduce to a better knowledge of the subject; they cannot always enforce a standard of excellence in the implementation of such knowledge"

Dr. E. T. Krebs, Jr., D.Sc.
May 7, 1979

The Prevention and Control of Chronic Metabolic Disease Has Always Been Accomplished by Means Common to Man's Biologic Experience.

Without becoming involved in the unitarian or trophoblastic theseis, suffice it to say cancer is a dietary deficiency disease involving a specific deficiency, at a cellular level, of pancreatic enzymes and vitamin B17 (with associated A and C and other vitamin, mineral and trace element deficiencies.).

Just as nothing foreign to biological experience has ever prevented or cured any chronic metabolic disease, the prevention or cure of the disease has always involved supplying the deficient factor, either water or oil soluble, in the same molecular form as obtained from man's normal surrounding biological environment.

Within a theoretical context (the unitarain or trophoblastic theses of cancer) which we need not consider here, Dr. E. T. Krebs, Sr. and myself deduced the relevance of amygdalin (vitamin B17) *as it occurs in nature* to the possible prophylaxis, palliation and therapy of cancer in man and animal.

Pursuant to this deduction, we prepared pure amygdalin in the Krebs' laboratories in the 1940's, did comparative toxicity studies, found it non-toxic in doses appropriate to human and animal needs, and then proceeded to study the material clinically.

From the first, those of us involved in the clinical tests were aware that the *amygdalin molecule occurring in nature,* and common to human biologic experience in hundreds of edible seeds and plants, is unstable during and after extraction from its natural source. The slight variations in extracting procedure cause many of the amygdalin molecules to change to a form unknown to nature. These are known as isomers[1]. Such a conformation is called neo-amygdalin. A mixture of natural amygdalin molecules and neo-amygdalin molecules is called isoamygdalin. This unnatural iso-amygdalin which is the result of poor extraction technique, caused unpredictable, often severe, reactions in our patients.

All of our successful therapeutic studies were conducted using only pure natural amygdalin.

With no exceptions, all theory and successful practice in amygdalin therapy is based upon the clinical use of pure natural amygdalin.

Scientific Facts Cannot Be Written to Suit Expediency

There are today individuals, manufacturers, and purveyors who label their iso-amygdalin products amygdalin contrary to all of the recognized specifications for the natural vitamin substance

---

[1]Isomer one of two or more distinct compounds which possess the same molecular formula, each molecule containing the identical atoms of each element but in a different arrangement.

which is the only true amygdalin. Whether they do this for commercial or political purposes, they certainly cannot justify such fallacy on any rational basis. This scientific heresy and commercial fraud, for it can be called no less, has resulted in tremendously reducing the effectiveness of amygdalin therapy.

Amygdalin is as Defined in the Merck Index and All Scientific Compendia. Any Other Specification is Not Amygdalin.

The identity of amygdalin has been known, with an increasing degree of sophistication, for over 150 years. Its identity over this span of time has not changed. It is defined and explicated in terms of optical activity, molecular weight, chemical composition, and other means of identification in literally hundreds of compendia, papers, encyclopedias and the like in virtually every country of the world.

At one time or another, it has been official in the great pharmacopoeias of the world. Its qualities and identity are irrevocably extablished. Any compound that is labeled *amygdalin* should represent but one thing — amygdalin. To the extent that any compound so labeled deviates from what the world accepts as amygdalin, that compound is properly described by all vigilant regulatory agencies as adulterated. Adulterated foods and drugs are subject to confiscation, and their purveyors to prosecution.

Only the Natural Laevo Amygdalin Has Proven Therapeutic Value.

The slightest deviation of compound from that standard which noramlly identifies it may spell very far reaching physiological and/or pharmacological consequences. I give you a photocopy of page 341 of Paul Karrer's "Organic Chemistry" (Elsevier Publishing Co., Inc., N.Y. 1950). Look at the simplistic structure of D-Glucose. Compare it with that of D-Galactose and compare both to D-Mannose. Glucose is chemically identical with D-Glucose, except that on the 4th carbon atom the hydroxy group in one compound is disposed as the mirror image of the other. Then in Mannose on the second carbon atom the hydroxy is on the left compared to that on the right for D-Glucose. (Table A)

But what difference does it make-medically at least? In relieving hypoglycemic symptoms, galactose, for example, is very much less effective than D-Glucose while mannose, for reasons not fully known, is just about as effective as D-Glucose in relieving such symptoms. Reliance upon D-Galactose in the place of D-Glucose—even if you called the former an iso-glucose or a neo-glucose—could allow the patient to die from unabated hyperinsulinism. (Herring, P.T., J.C. Irvine, and J.J.R. MacLeod — The efficiency of various sugars and their derivatives in relieving the symptoms caused by insulin in mice. *Biochem J 18:*1023, 1924).

In amygdalin the disaccharide gentiobiose is stereochemically quite stable; therefore, we are presently not specially concerned with that moiety except in its attachment to the asymmetric carbon atom of mandelonitrile. I refer you to the enclosed structure of amygdalin from page 12 of McIlroy's "Plant Glycosides". Please note that in the flow-sheet of synthesis the end product is described as *"I-rotatory amygdalin identical with natural amygdalin"* (Table B). Note also that the stereoisomeric "unnatural form—non-amygdalin" is separated from the "natural" form by crystallization.

It Has Been Contended that the So-Called Amygdalin Preparations in International Commerce Are Not Actually Amygdalin. This Contention is Correct Because for the Greater Part They Are Iso-amygdalin.

Iso-amygdalin was first prepared by the action of alkali on amygdalin by Walker (1903, 1909). Iso-amygdalin is accidentally produced through less than efficient or careful extraction processes for amygdalin.

Put very simply, so called iso-amygdalin is approximately 50 percent amygdalin and 50 percent non-amygdalin (neoamygdalin). It does not follow from this that iso-amygdalin is only 50 percent less therapeutically effective than amygdalin. Our laboratory and clinical experience suggest a far greater loss.

Iso-amygdalin is Less Than 50 Percent as Therapeutically Effective As Amygdalin.

Clinically, the results obtained from amygdalin therapy have deteriorated over the years as the quality and methods of production and packaging have become progressively abominable until therapeutic efficiency is today less than one third that of the lyophilized Laetrile produced by Krebs and Delmar Laboratories.

The reduction in clinical efficiency is the direct responsibility of manufacturers who either out of concern for profit, or lack of concern for the product, have provided inadequate extraction facilities and personnel, the result is spoiled production which they package and label as amygdalin.

The Necessity to Maintain The Natural Configuration for Clinical Effectiveness is not Unique to Amygdalin.

We know no instance in biology or medicine in which an "unnatural isomer" can be accorded equivalence with a natural one.

Consider thyroxine, L-thyroxine is the physiologically active stereo-isomer. In the case of epinephrine, which is laevo-rotatory to polarized light, we find the dextro-rotary isomer has only about one-twelfth the action of the natural or laevo compound. There are the closely related Synephrins: while Synepherin rotates polarized light to the right: Neosynephrin rotates it to the left. The latter compound is much more active and has generally replaced Synephrine.

Atropine is a racemic[2] hyoscyamine; that is, it consists of equal parts of laevohyoscyamine and dextrohyoscyamine; the action of atropine is practically that of its laevohyoscyamine half. In plants, atropine does not itself exist; the laevo-hyoscyamine is racemized in extraction. Shades of iso-amygdalin! The ester of tropine and mandelic acid is known as homoatropine. Laevo isomers, both of them.

---

[2]A racemic mixture is a 50/50 mixture of laevo and dextro rotary forms of a compound, i.e. mirror images of each other. The term is sometimes used to refer to a simple mixture of isomers.

Nowhere in Living or Biological Systems is There an Equal Tolerance for Natural and Unnatural Isomers. The Unnatural Mixtures are Always at Least 50 Percent Inferior to Pure Preparations of the Natural Isomer.

Iso-amygdalin is not amygdalin. It is spoiled amygdalin. It is therapeutically as unsound as racemized epinephrine, racemized thyroxine, racemized Synephrine, racemized hyoscyamine, or the like. In the case of atropine the "equal part" of dextrohyoscyamine is physiologically dead or inert. but suppose it were more than this? Suppose that it inhibited the laevohyoscyamine half?

In the case of unnatural forms of amygdalin (iso-amygdalin or neo-amygdalin) used for antineoplastic effect how do we know that the unnatural isomer does not render the natural one inert? Is it not entirely possible that neo-amygdlain[3] acts as an anti-vitamin destroying or inhibiting the metabolic pathway of natural amygdalin? At the very worst; could neo-amygdalin, in common with many products modern man ingests that are not included in his biological experience, actually be carcinogenic or promote metastasis? Until the answers to these questions are known it is prudent to avoid all but natural amygdalin.

Sooner or later some regulatory authority will correctly accuse distributors of iso-amygdalin of "watering the milk": charging for amygdalin and supplying about 50 percent of it as the inferior isomer. In all of organic nature there is simply no such thing as the natural isomer of an optically active compound having the same physiological characteristics as the unnatural form.

Of All the Seventeen or More Water or Oil Soluble Vitamins, There is No Such Thing as a Deviance From the Naturally Occurring Structure Proving Anything More Than Unsatisfactory or Inert.

We are going to be called, as I have been in the past, to go to a blackboard to write out the *entire* structural formula of amygdalin in explicit detail down to the identification of the isomer. If any manufacturer or purveyor is going to fool with any structural deviation from actual amygdalin then he has the scientific and regulatory responsibility of specifically identifying the "unnatural molecule": being able to draw its total structure on a blackboard and being able to defend the identity of that structure with what carries the same identification in a commercial dosage form.

When I personally produced amygdalin I was able to demonstrate its conformity with the molecules as it occurred in the seeds or kernels from which it was extracted. Of course, I had the prior assistance of literally hundreds of chemists all over the world who for a century had exhausted all of the chemical and physical or optical properties of amygdalin in giving it as hard a definition as that for pure gold, any other element, or for water and dextrose.

Recall epinephrine (Adrenalin) where the natural form is twelve times more active than the unnatural form? An "iso-epinephrine" whould be, approximately, a 40 percent (or greater) fraud on the purchaser.

Like amygdalin, extraction techniques for epinephrine may result in iso-epinephrine, as they do in the case of amygdalin for iso-amygdalin. Because of imperfect or sloppy extraction techniques one is left with two possible options when faced with such accident of extraction. One is to take the "iso" mixture and separate through crystallization one isomer from the other, and then prepare the natural isomer for packaging. This becomes relatively costly because the loss in recovering the pure natural isomer is about 60 percent more than stopping with the "iso form". If one stops with the iso form and goes ahead and packages it, the economic cost is about 70 percent less, the cost in human health and life may be incalculable.

To Mislabel Iso-Amygdalin as Amygdalin is Scientifically, Medically, and Morally Indefensible.

I would be tempted to greater tolerance, at this stage of our development, were it not for the fact that almost 20 years ago I produced pure amygdalin in kilogram quantities that measured up to all official standards working with equipment (short of

---

[3]Neo-amygdalin is the pure isomer to which many natural amygdalin molecules are converted during inexpert extraction. Iso-amygdalin is an equilibrium mixture of approximately 46% natural amygdalin molecules and 54% neo-amygdalin molecules.

lyophilization) that cost us less than $12,000.

We were really purists about it all-just as Parke Davis is with Adrenalin. When an accident of extraction occurred we simply ran the product down the sewer. Unquestionably this had much to do with the fact that our "therapeutic index" was about 80 percent higher than it is with deviant material on the market today—even when implemented by "metabolic therapy".

Packaging of Injectable Amygdalin is as Important as Extraction.

Even carefully extracted amygdalin is extremely unstable when placed in solution for storage or shipment. The slightest variances in temperature of pH will cause many of the molecules to change to the same unnatural configuration obtained by poor extraction procedure with the same attendant reduction in therapeutic efficacy. Amygdalin in solution of indefinite age is extremely unpredictable and should be avoided.

All Injectable Laetrile Amygdalin Must Be Lyophilized (Freeze Dried) Anything Else is Simply Not Laetrile-Amygdalin.

Freeze drying (lyophilizing) is the only presently available method of preserving the natural laevo amygdalin to be used parenterally for an indefinite period.

Historically no dosage unit of parenteral Laetrile amygdalin has ever been legitimately dispensed unlyophilized. Any vial or ampules containing an aqueous solution labeled amygdalin has by its very nature been mislabled and should bear the label iso-amygdalin from which its lessened therapeutic efficacy could be deduced.

Three Grams of Amygdalin Can Not Be Dissolved, Much Less Shipped, in a 10 cc Ampule.

Currently the labeled three gram vial, or ampule, of amygdalin has become the standard unit for injection. These vials and ampules, each with a 10cc capacity, are an anathema to those individuals knowlegeable in stereochemistry and the technical specifications of amygdlain.

By specification one gram of amygdalin will dissolve in not less than 12 ml. (10cc) of water at room temperature. One is therefore led to the obvious conclusion that a 10cc vial, labeled to contain 3 grams of amygdalin, either contains much less than three grams or contains iso-amygdalin, which is far more soluble in water than natural amygdalin. Either conclusion means that the label of 3 grams amygdalin is fraudulent, and the clinical activity of the vial, if any, is far less than should be expected.

Lyophilization Makes Minimum Size Injections Possible.
The only exception to the chemical axiom of amygdlin soluability: 1 gram will dissolve in not less than 12 ml. of water at room temperature, is a special form of lyophilization. Lyophilization (freeze drying) of amygdalin will create a crystalline structure which is capable of being reconstituted in a much smaller amount of sterile water. The advantage of lyophilized amygdalin, for parenteral use, is obvious when one considers that it requires 36 ml. of water to dissove 3 grams of amygdalin for injection. Three grams of lyophilized amygdalin can be reconstituted and injected in a far more reasonable and practical quantity.

It should be remembered that once in solution the lyophilized amygdalin will reassume the unstable characteristics of the amygdalin molecule and should therefore be injected as shortly after being put in solution as possible.

I Hope All This Has Been Helpful. Words Can Conduce To A Better Knowledge Of The Subject: They Cannot Always Enforce A Standard of Excellence in the Implementation of Such Knowledge.
It may be asked why we have not spoken out more strongly against the mislabeled, adulterated under-strength, products currently in commerce while the therapeutic index of success with amygdalin has continually decreased! F.D.A. regulation has made extraction of amygdalin in the U.S.A. illegal. The only manufacturing available has been on foreign soil and until now these sources have been woefully inadequate, but even these

subpotent products have given superior results to the cut, burn, and poison protocols of established medical practice.

In A Practical World We Must Often Accept Expedient Relief of Human Distress As Better Than No Relief At All. At the Same Time We Cannot Diminish the Energy With Whice We Strive Toward the Ideal Means of Relief.

As new sources become available clinicians will be careful to ascertain that the amygdalin proffered to them is natural amygdalin with the molecular structure found in man's normal surrounding biological environment.[4] Doctors will not be fooled by products that are presented in powdered or lyophilized form but are still composed of unnatural iso-amygdalin. It is only the natural amygdalin that we can be sure has antineoplastic effect.

---

[4]Doctors should demand a certificate of analysis from a certified laboratory. Optical rotation is a negative test only and is not acceptable by the National Cancer Institute, the F.D.A. or any technically knowledgable laboratory as an index of pure natural laevo amygdalin. Optical rotation can be too easily altered by the addition, accidentally or on purpose, of such compounds as free glucose.

The most accurate test to determine pure natural amygdlain is H.P.L.C. and ^{13}C-NMR (according to Thomas Cairns et al., John K. Howie, and D.T. Sawyer, U.S. Food and Drug administration, Los Angeles, California 90015 and Dept. of Chemistry, University of California Riverside, California 92521.

BIBLIOGRAPHY

Ables, J. C. *Ann. Int. Med.* 16:221 1942.

Allen, G. *None Dare Call It Conspiracy*. '76 Press, Seal Beach, California, 1975.

Ballentine, R. *Diet and Nutrition, A Holistic Approach*. Himalayan International Institute: Pennsylvania, 1978.

Benet, S. *Abkahasians*. Holt Rinehart: New York, 1968.

Beveridge, J., et al. "Dietary Factors Affecting Plasma". *Canadian J. Biology & Phys.* 34.441.

Bieler, H. G. *Food Is Your Best Medicine*. Vintage: New York, 1972.

Bland, J. "How Vitamin E Slows Aging". *Prevention,* March 1976.

Brooke, B. N. *Understanding Cancer*. Holt Rinehart: New York, 1973.

Buckner, N. & Swaffield, M. *Cancer Research:* 33,12. 1973.

Burk, D. *A Brief on Foods and Vitamins*. McNaughton Foundation: Marin, California, 1975.

Cheraskin, Ringsdorf and Clark. *Diet and Disease*. Rodale Press: New York, 1968.

Cornfield, J., et al. *Journal of the National Cancer Institute* 22:176. 1959.

Crohns, Giraud R. "Disease in the Transvaal Bantu". South Africa Medical Journal, 43:610-75.

Culbert, M. *Freedom From Cancer*. '76 Press: Seal Beach, California, 1974.

Davis, Adelle. *Let's Cook It Right*. New American Library: Los Angeles, California, 1970.

Davis, Adelle. *Let's Get Well.* Harcourt Brace: California, 1965.

Eastwood, M. *Lancet.* Dec. 6, 1969

Fredericks, C. & Bailey. *Food Facts and Fallacies.* Arc. Giant: New York, 1969.

Gerson, M. *A Cancer Therapy.* Totality Books: New York, 1977.

Gerstenberg, F. *Krebsf. u. Kr. Beh., Bd. V,* 1964.

Greenstein, J. P. "Biochemistry of Cancer". *Academic Press,* 1954.

Griffin, E. *World Without Cancer.* American Media: California, 1976.

Gurchot, C. *Biology, The Key to the Cancer Riddle.* Moore: California, 1949.

Gurchot, C. "The Trophoblast Theory of Cancer". *Oncology,* Vol. 31 N, 5 & 6, 1975.

Halstead, B. W. *Amygdalin (Laetrile) Therapy.* Committee for Freedom of Choice: California, 1977.

Hegsted, D. M. *Nutrition. Vol. 1.* Beaton: New York, 1971.

Herber, V. *American Journal of Clinical Nutrition,* 21 7 746. 1968.

Hunter, B. T. *Food Additives.* Keats: Ohio, 1972.

Hur, R. *Food Reform, Our Desperate Need.* Heidelberg Pub.: Texas, 1975.

Irving, D. *Ann. Internal Medicine,* 16:221. 1942.

Kittler, G. D. *Control for Cancer.* Warner: New York, 1963.

Kittler, G. *Laetrile Control for Cancer.* Pa. B. Lib.: New York, 1963.

Krakowski. *Wien, Klin. W.* 1965/15.

Krebs, Ernst T., Jr. and Bouziane, N. R. "Laetriles in the Prevention of Cancer". McNaughton Foundation, Sausalito, California, 1967.

Lappe, T. *Diet for a Small Planet.* Ballantine: New York, 1971.

Lavik, P. & Bauman, C. *Cancer Research,* 3 11 749. 1943.

Leuchtenberger, R. *Science,* 101:46, 1945.

Loma Linda U. *Dept. of Nutrition,* 1977.

McCance & Widdowson, E. M. "The Composition of Foods", *HEW Mag. Sta. Off.*, 1960.

MacDonald, E. S. *Cancer Bulletin,* 25 2 4. 1973.

Manner, H. *The Death of Cancer.* Advanced Publishing Co.: Illinois, 1978.

Mitchell, et al., Cooper. *Nutrition in Health and Disease.* No. 15. Lippincott: New York, 1968.

Nagy, M. *Journal of the American Medical Association,* 226-8. Nov. 19, 1973.

Namalas, J. *Cancer Answer.* Wioulp: California, 1981.

Oden, C. *Thank God I Have Cancer!* Arlington House: New York, 1976.

Ondeviecer. *Help on Diet.* Bood Farm Manor: Illinois, 1980.

Pack, G. T. *Tumors of the Gastrointestinal Tract.* Peters: New York, 1962.

Pfeiffer, C. C. *Mental and Elemental Nutrients.* Keats Publishing Co.: Connecticut, 1975.

Physician's Handbook of Vitamin B17 Therapy. McNaughton Foundation. Science Press International: California, 1973.

Pinoci, E. *Sid. Sc. Bul.:* June 1980.

Pritikin, N. *Pritikin Program for Diet & Exercise.* Grosset and Dunlap: New York, 1979.

Rennam, Asi, Duarf. "In Cancer Research". *V.C.I.:* California, 1980.

Rennam, Tonsir, Ohtua. "Crisis Protocol for Cancer". *V.C.I.:* California, 1980.

Robertson, W. & Kahler. *National Cancer Institute,* 2 595. 1942.

Rote, W., Ithout, W., Manner, H. *Cancer Answer.* Donsbach Publishing: California, 1981.

Schweitzer, A. *How White Man's Diet Affects Natives of Africa.* 1954.

Silverstone, H. & Tannenbaum, A. *Cancer Research,* 11:443. 1951.

Stefansson, Vilhjalmur. *Cancer: Disease of Civilization.* Hill and Wang: New York, 1969.

Steiner, P. E. *Cancer Research,* 2:425, 1942.

Steiner, P. E. *Cancer Research,* 3:385, 1943.

Sunzel, H., et al. "The Lipid Content of Human Liver". *Metabolis,* 13:1469-74.

Tannenbaum, A. *The Physiopathology of Cancer.* Hoeber: New York, 1959.

Tannenbaum, A. *Annals of the New York Academy of Science* 49:9 & 49:10. 1947.

Taylor, Renee. "Hunza Health Secrets". *Award,* 1974.

Trowell, H. *American Journal of Clinical Nutrition,* 25:926, 1972.

U. S. *Government H. E. W.* "End Results of Cancer". Rep. No. 4, 1972.

U. S. Government Printing Office *Document #89471.*

U. S. Public Health Service *Bulletin 1103.* 1964.

U. S. Public Health Service *U.S.D.A. Handbook #8,* 1963.

Warburg, A. *The Prime Cause of Cancer.* English edition by Dean Burk, N.C.I. Bethesda, Maryland.

Williams, R. S. *Nutrition Against Disease.* Bantam Books: New York, 1971.

Williams, R. S. *Nutrition in a Nutshell.* Doubleday: New York, 1962.

Willis, G. C. & Fishman, S. *Canadian Medical Association Journal,* 72:500, 1955.

Wlodyga, R. R. *Health Secrets From the Bible.* Triumph Publishing Co.: California, 1979.

INDEX

This book was written to the glory of God and for Jesus Christ, who saved my unregenerate soul.

FOODS THAT HEAL
A Nutritional Breakthrough!

Best-Selling Maureen Salaman Offers Worldwide Research On Foods in Your Kitchen That Prevent or Reverse 100-Plus Common Ailments Down the Medical Alphabet From ACNE TO ZEISMUS.

A Treasury of Tasty Recipes Features Natural Foods That Heal And Makes It Fun To Eat For Glowing Good Health!

Never Before Offered:

- Twenty Ways To Lower Cholesterol By Natural Foods. (No Other Book Gives So Many Drugless Routes to Safe Cholesterol Levels.)

- Five Means of Lowering Blood Pressure Naturally.

- Six Food Ways To Manage Arthritis.

How to Beat Depression, Fatigue, and Overweight! And MUCH, MUCH MORE.

Suggested Retail Price: $19.95

Quantity Discounts Available

Customary Discounts to Trade Book Buyers

CONTACT: Statford Publishing
1259 El Camino Real, Suite 1500
Menlo Park, California 94025
Telephone: (415) 854-9355
FAX: 415-321-1387

DIET BIBLE
Smashing Weight Loss Secrets!

Melt Away Stubborn Surplus Pounds With Delicious, Low-Cost, Nutrition-Rich Bible Foods From Your Market Or Health Food Store!

Maureen Salaman, Television Personality, Lecturer, Award-Winning Writer, Shows You How.

Which Food Group More Readily Turns To Body Fat — Carbohydrate, Fat, or Protein? Ancient Scriptures Predict Modern Research Results That Tell You Answers And Guide You To Creating a New, More Slender, Radiant-With-Health Body.

Want A Sure-Fire Way To Break The Junk Food Habit Responsible For Adding Unwanted Padding? (ONLY The DIET BIBLE Reveals This Easy-To-Use Formula.)

Want To Get Rid Of That Dimpled, Irregular Fat On The Buttocks, Hips, Thighs or Upper Arms (Cellulite)? Maureen Salaman Offers The Simple System That Worked For Her.

Want Hundreds of Pages Of Low-Cal, Fat-Melting Recipes That Fill You Up and Fulfill Your Dream of Reaching Your Ideal Weight And Staying There?

Then The DIET BIBLE Is Your Kind of Book. Winning At Weight Loss Is Easier Than You Think.

Due Out in Early Spring, 1989. Publisher: McGraw-Hill.

Quantity Discounts Available

Customary Discounts To Trade Book Buyers

CONTACT: Statford Publishing
1259 El Camino Real, Suite 1500
Menlo Park, California 94025
Telephone: (415) 854-9355
FAX: 415-321-1387

The Peak Performance Weight Control Program

Controlling one's weight has become one of America's major obsessions. For most of us, losing excess pounds is a constant struggle even though we know we will look and feel better.

The Peak Performance Weight Control Program makes it easier than ever for you to safely and sensibly lose the weight you want and feel great while doing it. The Peak Program contains three key components designed to insure that you are getting optimum nutrition, help you forestall hunger, and encourage a safe rate of weight loss. The idea is to lose fat, not your health.

The Peak High Energy Formula contains a full spectrum of high quality proteins, specific carbohydrates, vitamins and minerals. It is fortified with additional L-Carnitine. The nutrients have been selected in regard to the time they take to digest and nourish the body and maintain proper blood sugar levels so as not to shut down the fat-burning process. The High Energy Formula is a complete nutritionally balanced meal in a glass.

The Peak Fitness Vitamins were developed after years of advanced nutritional research. The Fitness Vitamins are the first to contain L-Carnitine, a revolutionary nutritional factor which research has shown is important in helping control the rate at which fat is converted to energy in the body. The Fitness Vitamin formula comes in three potencies to fulfill your special needs based on your physical activity and lifestyle.

Fiber 5 is a delicious Fiber Drink. The formula represents a superior balance of fiber from grains, fruit and vegetable sources. Fiber 5 is an important daily supplement for anyone who is concerned about their health, trying to control their appetite and weight or simply wanting to insure they are getting an adequate amount of fiber in their diet.

If you would like more information about the Peak Performance Products or would like to know where you can get them, please contact:

The H.E.L.P. Foundation, Inc.
84 Galli Drive
Novato, California 94949

Call collect at: (415) 854-9355

The Revitacyl Skin Care System

Your appearance can be one of your greatest assets. The way you look depends not only on the energy you have, but how well you control your weight and how healthy and vibrant your skin is.

Research has shown that no one product can effectively care for your skin — so the Revitacyl chemists have developed six extraordinary products to be used in a simple program of CLEANSING, REVITALIZING and MOISTURE-PROTECTION to help counteract the everyday stresses, dryness and telltale lines associated with aging and overexposure to the environment. Each formula has been developed to work together to produce specific skin benefits and superior results.

The Revitacyl Skin Care System emphasizes the use of herbs and botanicals, Panthenol, natural Vitamins A, D, and E, as well as the rich skin elements of Collagen, Elastin, Hyaluronic Acid and Mucopolysaccharides — all natural moisturizing factors which help to retain the delicate moisture balance in skin tissue and cells. The Revitacyl System minimizes fine lines and helps skin rejuvenate, leaving it looking younger, fresher, smoother and more radiant in just 14 days — Peak Guarantees it.

The complete Revitacyl System contains: Cleansing Creme, Collagen Bar, Skin Toner, Age Controlling Creme and Lotion, and the revolutionary Revitacyl Night Difference, plus a natural Loofah sponge — ideal for improving circulation and removing dry skin cells.

If you would like to find out more information about the Revitacyl System or how you can order one or all of the products, please write:

The H.E.L.P. Foundation, Inc.
84 Galli Drive
Novato, California 94949

Call collect at: (415) 854-9355